If I offend anyone with my vulgarity or lascivious behavior, I apologize. Actually I don't. Go fuck yourself. As my grandpa always told me, be yourself Chris. Vaya Con Dios Grandpa!

The information contained in this book is based upon the research and personal and professional experience of the author. It is not intended as a substitute for consulting with your physician or other healthcare provider. Any attempt to diagnose and treat an illness should be done under the direction of a healthcare professional. This book is intended as a reference volume only, not as a medical manual. The information given here is designed to help you make informed decisions on your health, diet, fitness, and exercise program aka S.P.I.N.E.™. It is not intended as a substitute for medical advice. If you suspect that you have a medical problem, I urge you to seek competent medical attention. As with all exercise programs, you should seek your doctors approval before you begin. You will not hold the VTD or Show Up Fitness, LLC liable for any claims, demands, injuries, damages, actions or causes of action, whatsoever, to my person or property arising out of or connected with actions from the VTD. I agree to abide by the recommendations of my physician when embarking on my new exercise program.

Mention of specific companies, organizations, or authorities in this book does not imply endorsements nor does mention of specific companies, organizations, or authorities imply that they endorse this book. Internet addresses given in this book were accurate at the time it went to press.

Editors: Michael J. Hitchko & Magen Petit
Cover design: Jaime Verab www.bidesignllc.com
Images within book: Durer remake: Louise Poulso from London, United Kingdom.
Hormone Cartoons (Hormone Glossary Only): Tyrus Goshay & Nicholas Callow, Chicago, Illinois.
All other images: Hallow Graphics
All artists were located via www.guru.com

Exercise Photo's: Robert Silver @ www.getlivemedia.com
Additional credit to Laura Silverman for editing help with Chapters 5&6.
Printed in the United States of America.

Table of contents

Acknowledgements

I dedicate this book to my brothers, parents and Alexa. We are a unique group and not many understand our bond. It's who we are and I love you all for it (all Hitchkos and Schmitz included.) It's the one thing that will always be here for us no matter the circumstances. Mom and Pops you two are the most patient, smart people I know. Thanks for life and giving us the best upbringing any kids could ask for. I will always be indebted to you. Hopefully this book hits it big time and I can buy you guys that ranch away from all the crazy people in the world. Hitchkos' four life.

My amazingly beautiful and supportive girlfriend. Thanks for putting up with Jacko, my brothers, guys night and me. We are unique, that's for damn sure and you are super patient and awesome. 5683.

To my editors Magen Petit and Dr. Commander Hitchko. Your patience and guidance is unparalleled. Dad, you have made my blabber into a 260+ page book!!! You only spent 600 hours editing it, it was worth it, right?

Jaime Verab for all the graphic design help and confidence boosting during our days at UCONN!

Dr. Kraemer, though you will probably never read this, you'll always be my number one man crush and always will be.

Brie and Melissa at Dublin Transition. Working with your students keeps me grounded and a better, more appreciative person. You two are awesome teachers.

David Tweed. Without you, I wouldn't be where I am today writing this book, literally. That night you came into the classroom and gave me that God awful book on weight loss (which I ended up losing, whoops) motivated me to write this. That book you gave me was so fucking boring and misleading; I almost blew my brains out. Luckily I didn't because I ended up writing this masterpiece! You're an awesome trainer.

Students who've challenged me.

My beautiful models who were patient with me and took the photos for the exercise chapter: Lindsey, Leah and Kaseena. All three of them graduated from my personal training program. They're perfect examples of practicing what they preach. Additionally, they're trainers for my company Show Up Fitness- I only hire the best! Thanks ladies!

Penises. As I love to draw you on the back of dirty car windows and bathroom windows.

Boobs. As I want to stick my face between every pair I see.

Sex. As you are the coolest thing on this earth.

Dogs. For being the best creatures on this earth.

To most of my Ex-girlfriends. Thanks for the fuel to fire my diatribes. I hope you all languish in your genital warts and I wish for a continual cloud of pigeon shit to fall on your head.

Jackson, I hope a pack of wolves eats you on your next hunting trip.

Love, joy, peace, patience, kindness, goodness, happiness, faithfulness and self-control.

RIP: Grandpa's, Grandma's, Miles, Kit, Bobbie, and Pendleton and Doug.

About Me:

My name is Chris Hitchko. I grew up in Chico, California. I learned how to throw water balloons at fat cops and received a minor in alcoholism.   I was a tad chubby, but that was because I took so much Prednisone to manage my chronic bronchitis and a cluster of other shitty ailments. I had Mono, Hay Fever, Asthma and Gonorrhea; you name it, I had it. Wait a second, I had Giardia - I knew it started with a G. Regardless, my mom thought I was a cute kid. As we all know, there are no sympathy points with the ladies. Let's be honest mom, I was a fat ass. I was always busy with sports, trying to kick some ass, but experienced some injuries. I claim it was from the antibiotics and Prednisone, but doctors said it wasn't. I still believe that I should be a 6-foot-6 starting shooting guard in the NBA. Just let me hang onto that one. With the NBA out the window, I decided on physical therapy. I figured I could help young kids get stronger and prevent injuries. I graduated with a degree in Kinesiology from California State University, Chico. During my undergrad, I completed a year at the University of Connecticut as an exchange student. At both Universities, I learned from some of the most spectacular minds in Kinesiology and Nutrition. I decided to continue my education and become a Certified Strength and Conditioning Specialist (CSCS), which is regarded as the highest certification in the personal training industry.   I'm not tooting my own horn, but I do know a lot about exercise and nutrition. Let's make it perfectly clear that there are many individuals who know more about these topics than I do, I am just delivering the information in a new and fun way. I will always admit when I am wrong and continually inspire to learn more. This shit will continue to amaze me!

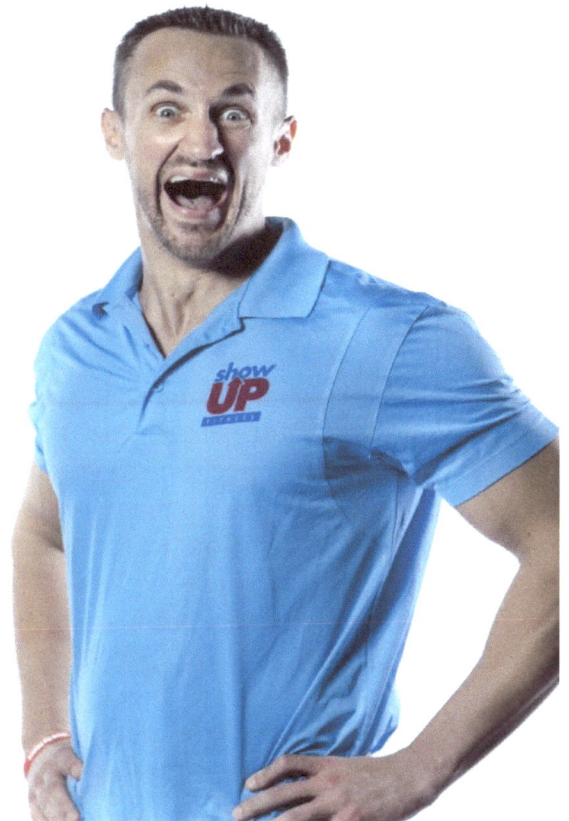

After graduation, I wasn't sure what I wanted to be when/if I grew up. I needed money badly so I could pay off my student loans. Hmmm what to do; Thunder Down Under stripper here I come! I could have, which would have made for a better story, but I became a Personal Trainer in the San Francisco Bay Area instead. I loved training. Clients, who were dedicated and listened were amazing - the results showed. The ones who complained and didn't follow through were still fat and out of shape. People are full of excuses or plain and simple, just a bunch of pussies. How do you think you are going to get the results you desire if you don't Show Up? Excuses are the easy way out and people are constantly searching for them. So, after five years of training, I was fortunate enough to start working as an instructor at a personal training school.   The program is six months in length reviewing hundreds of hours in anatomy, physiology, biochemistry, biomechanics, and hands-on training to gain experience. My boss is awesome. She lives in LA and never comes up to the Bay Area, where the school is located. I hold the reins and do what I do best, teach while helping those who want to learn.

In October 2011, I started my own personal training company, Show Up Fitness (hence all the Show Up references - it's such a catchy phrase, but don't worry, there will be many more to come). During my tenure, I have worked with professional athletes, old folks, young kids, people wanting to lose weight, gain weight, youngsters, and teens with special needs and everything in-between.

Show Up Fitness opened as a result of me observing clients whose failures resided from not showing up regularly. Under my instruction, clients would learn about exercise, fat loss, dieting, and even tidbits on relationships, sex, and love. Maybe they needed some prodding and guidance about proper form. BAM! Results would be achieved for those who showed up. However, those who used excuses and missed training sessions because they were too tired or overwhelmed, were excluded and never achieved their results. The gravy train to fat land held a ticket with their name on it and guess who they wanted to blame? Yeah, I am the 'bad trainer' because they were the "Kings and Queens of Excuses." Tough love people; it's your own fucking fault! This reminds me of the story about the married couple who went to see a counselor. The counselor wanted to start the session off in a positive fashion, so he asked, "What do you two have in common?" And the husband replied, "Neither of us likes to give blow jobs!" Where was I going with that? Oh well, I guess it will come to me later.

Show Up
Why do you think people lose weight from doing high intense programs that you see on TV? They demand that the person exercises 5-6 times a week. It isn't hard to get results if you are doing a high intensity program five times a week. I wonder where all the people are who hurt themselves from overuse injuries and too many repetitions? That's the problem with these programs, they are not for everyone. What about the obese and debilitated individuals who cannot perform these high intensity exercises? They are left behind for further injuries and never heard from again. In my opinion, these workouts are sub-par, designed improperly, and the instructors are outrageously annoying. Well it's time to listen to someone who actually knows what they are talking about. Implement this awesomely fantastic system and you'll soon discover what it feels like to achieve greatness! These workouts will get you the results you have wanted for years because I will teach you how to exercise properly. You will no longer feel like a robot following people like you're in "Thriller" music video. The days of spending hours pussy farting around the gym and doing cardio for two hours are over. Dieting will be easier than ever. You will learn what to eat, when and how much. You are going to transform your body into something amazing! Cheat foods and meals will be allowed because your metabolism will be able to handle it. Your energy levels and sex drive will shoot through the roof. Stress levels will subside and your overall outlook toward life will be heightened. This book will be your Bible for total health. I will teach you how to get those washboard abs like mine (sorry not a braggart, just the truth), lose those flabby arms, and get rid of the infamous beer gut. Also, I'll help you identify how many days you should be training and if your goals are even realistic by using the S.P.I.N.E.™ Questionnaire.

Chapter 1

Intro to S.P.I.N.E.™:

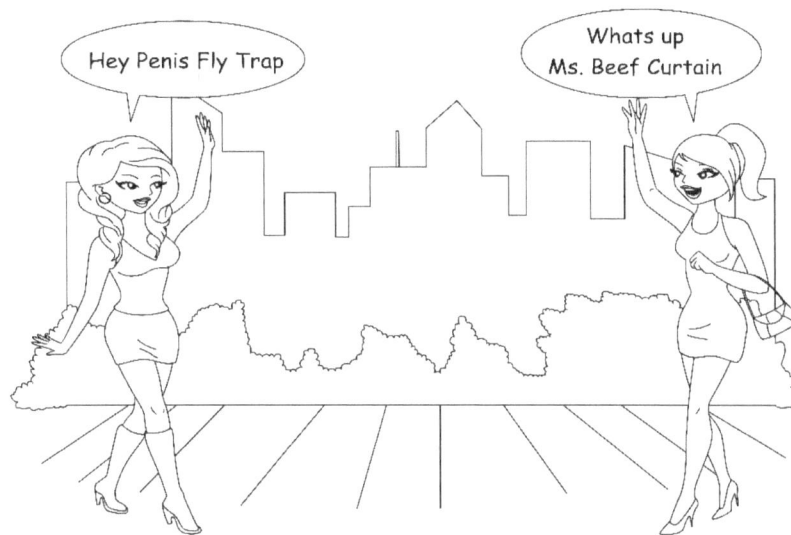

The Vulgar Truth Diet aka VTD, is not an STD; it's a fitness constitution. This book will teach you about exercise, nutrition, and how to manage stressors. We've created the best pill in the world to combat fatness; it's called exercise. Ironically, the government and pharmaceutical companies are trying to create a pill that replaces the hard work necessary with exercise. This is where we have gone wrong. We are looking for drugs to fix everything. I know where the answer lies; it's in the acronym S.P.I.N.E.™: Sex, Stress, Sleep, Psychology, Injuries, Nutrition, and Exercise. Addressing all seven aspects will turn realistic goals into something tangible.

My goal is to teach you how to fix it. In order to make it in this industry, it's necessary to ruffle some feathers; so let the ruffling begin! This book is not a magical serum or a collection of fancy fake terms like "muscle confusion" and "muscle memory." It's an honest attempt on the "how-to" get yourself into the greatest shape of your life. The best part of getting there is no crazy diet or counting calories or any sales pitch!

I was taught in school that most diets and programs are shitty because they're anecdotal. That's the thing; VTD is a system, not a program. Programs need a follow up and usually fail. Systems are for a lifetime. A lot of inaccurate information is being spread by trainers and "experts" who are just "spouting off" without the benefit of scientific evidence. I'll just stick to my scientific background, sailor's vocabulary, and amazing beard. At times, my father disputes my verbiage and feels that I should be more succinct - fairly easy to say for a former English teacher and Ph.D. in Counseling Psychology. It's not that I can't be an erudite; I can throw some fancy words at you any day of the week. Sometimes I feel it's easier to say fucking donkey shit, rather than, "I am thoroughly displeased with that decision." Let's just go with there's always a time and a place, or as one chick once told me, "Know your audience." – Man, I miss her big fake boobs.

Honestly, there are a lot of falsehoods, and, even flat out lies that saturate our fitness society. Call me old-fashioned, but I believe trainers should be educated; most are not, they're egotistical idiots. The majority of personal trainers today go online and take a 100- to 200-question exam - within a matter of a few weeks (sometimes days), they're certified personal trainers. How crazy is that! I live by the motto, "Teach first, train second." I was motivated to write this book because most books on exercise and nutrition are esoteric piles of kangaroo shit, not to mention boring. The material can be interesting if you're able to decipher it, but the average person, is lost from the get go. I am a proponent of scientific literature; however, my students and clients agree that it's like pulling teeth to understand. Some of the best places to look and find scientific information are textbooks – boring! Try reading a few pages before bed and that's more soporific than the best sleeping pill! I am going to bring valid information to the "bro-science" community in a fun, entertaining way. One of my skills is teaching difficult material in an understanding, sometimes makeshift, yet, fun way! You are going to laugh, be offended, and inspired to workout in the proper manner. This book is for males and females. Young and old. Skinny and fat. Horny and, you get the point, it's for any human body. We need to understand that sexy abs, defined arms, nice legs, an awesome ass, and a strong back are earned! Sometimes, everyone needs a cowboy boot in their ass; be it a large, medium, or small sized one! And, this book will be the cowboy boot in the ass!

What to Expect
Don't you hate it when you watch a trailer for a movie and it totally looks like it's going to rock only to discover when you watch the movie it's worse than the smell of a baboon's ass? Spoiler alert! I'm going to tell you exactly what to expect in this book. If one of these 11 reasons doesn't work for you, don't buy it. You'll just end up bitching and putting bad reviews on Yelp or Amazon and ain't nobody got time for that!

The Good Expectations
1. How to fix your S.P.I.N.E.™. As a result, you'll achieve greater energy levels, self-confidence, a better body, a new wardrobe, smiles, laughter, and loving yourself. Now, for the infomercial pitch... Fuck that! It may sound corny, but when we fix your S.P.I.N.E.™, all of this will happen.

2. Debunking misconceptions. Ladies, you won't turn into the Hulk and get big and bulky. Guys, you won't grow a vagina if you do some cardio. Eating before bed won't make your happy parts fall off and turn you into Pizza-The-Hut. All carbs aren't bad. Saturated fats won't kill you. Soy actually is the devil. I'll be your Huckleberry and debunk the shit out of things you hear all day long with no validity to their claims.

3. Trendy, with the best of the old. The VTD is like Randy Houser and Garth Brooks. Oh shit, I forgot that people don't listen to country music. How about Katy Perry and Michael Jackson? The exercise

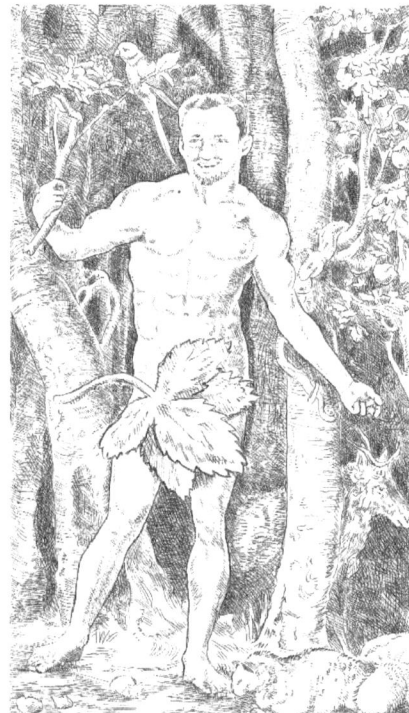

workouts will be based on undulating periodization (fancy word for changing the rep scheme per workout.) The VTD diet plan will follow a grain-free diet with the addition of nutrient timing, fasting, and detoxing, all in one. The best part is there will be no counting kcals. Together, we will change your behaviors to help teach you how to make better choices.

4. Learning and laughter. I'm a teacher and I'm good at what I do. You will learn a crap load about exercise, nutrition, injuries, history, and why I am bat shit crazy. I will make fun of a lot of people including myself so don't worry. You think I would put a redrawing of Albrecht Durer's *Adam and Eve* painting on the cover because I thought it was cool? No. I'm making fun of myself (look at my effeminate pose) and the people who actually do that shit! Ohhhh Narcissism.

5. Lots of sexuality. Who doesn't like sex? You're probably crazy because you aren't having enough of it! If you're like my brother Mike and can go without it, so be it. Otherwise, I'm a man's man and make bold sexual statements, be prepared.

6. No stupid fucking weird-ass exercises. If you want to stay fat, then continue performing those bizarre exercises that you see in magazines, DVD's or infomercials! Most exercises that you need to do in the confines of your own home (minus having your own gym), probably means it won't do jack shit. You'd be better off sticking your thumb up your ass - that would probably yield better results!

The Bad Expectations (depending on how you look at it...) *please pay close attention to numbers 7 & 8. I believe this book is for everybody, but realistically, the age range of 18-45. My mommy always told me honesty is the best policy!*

7. I am not sensitive. I grew up with brothers and have always practiced tough love - deal with it. I will not sympathize with your excuses. If you're *fat, you're fat - get over it. The opportunity to change is within this book, and the choice is yours. Are you going to continue to bitch and tell the world why you suck? No sympathy here. You're better off trying to get some sympathy votes by squatting on a cactus. If you listen to everything I have to say and Show Up, you'll be a changed person. *I call everyone and everything fat in a fun loving way, you'll soon realize, it's the Hitchko sarcasm.

8. Vulgarity and crass drawings. This book will insult the FUCK out of you if the following words are offensive: Fuck, shit, dickface, asshole, pussy-fart, fucktard and/or any synonyms for: fuck, shit, pussy, dickface, asshole, pussy-fart, and fucktard so get the fuck over it! If vulgar language isn't your cup of tea, fuck off.

9. Ignorance vs Stupidity. As I tell my students, if you are unaware of something, that's ignorance; adapt and improve. Implement the new idea to see for yourself. This shit works. If you go back to your old methods that haven't worked, then, you're stupid. Einstein said it best, "You're a fucking moron if you do the same damn thing over and over again and expect different results." Did I misquote that?

10. Sense of humor. If you're boring and can't understand that I am trying to relay information in a fun and entertaining way...see number 8.

11. The Truth. Hence the name of the book, it's the truth and some won't like it. People will be offended and not commit 100%, that's why you'll stay unsatisfied with your body image. I honestly wish you the best with your future endeavors, but this book isn't for you.

12. I am human. I have gathered this information by corroborating 10 years of personal training, coaching basketball and track, all of the courses that I took in college, reading countless books, continuing education classes, and professionals I have met. With that being said, some of the shit I say may be incorrect - or as my dad says, logorrhea. That's the wonderful thing about life, you live and you learn. By the time you finish reading this book, I will already be a better teacher with new information that I have learned.

The one thing I won't do is feed you shit, make false promises, or sell you on something that isn't achievable. It will not be easy, but it will be rewarding. To achieve success, you need to encounter discomfort (write that down - 10-1 odds that quote will be in a calendar someday). Everyone's life is filled with stress. Family issues arise. Divorces happen. Kids stress us out. You shit your pants next to that hot girl in class. We all have been there. Just because you throw an excuse out there, doesn't mean I care. In the end, if you want the results, listen to what I have to say, bottom line. Yes, I have a heart and no, I wasn't raised by just my dad. My mom is an angel; literally, I don't know how she raised us. Four boys and my dad had to be tough, but I used her compassion to help write this. Life is challenging for everyone. You are given the decision to Show Up and give it 100% or look for excuses and settle for mediocrity. "No man has the right to be an amateur in the matter of physical training. It is a shame for a man to grow old without seeing the beauty and strength of which his body is capable" – Socrates. Socrates basically just said Show Up or Shut the Fuck UP! Remember, its pronounced So-Crates (from Bill and Ted's- C'MON!)

Now, the choice is yours. You can change your current lifestyle and be happy forever, or, you can be a coward and look for that quick fix (we both know that it will eventually come back and bite you in your fat ass). Listen to my words and you'll be a fat-loss winner. If you stray, it's ok, get back on the VTD plan. I will teach you how to beat fat conclusively. And, the best part? You will be the one who earned it! No more excuses; the time is now. Buckle down, grab a bottle of whiskey, and ask yourself this question: are you ready to Show Up?

How to fix your S.P.I.N.E.™? Begin here by implementing these 5 new things each week:
Sex - If you're not having some sort of sexual interaction at least *3 – 4x a week, you're 2x as likely to get hit by a car and/or die a horrible death. Ok, that's not true, but something needs to scare the holy shit out of you to start humping more! Shoot for 3x this week. No stupid fucking excuses either. Sex is probably one of the coolest things on this earth (besides my beard). How about a morning quickie? Or some wet and naughty fun in the shower. It's easy to clean up and the kids can't bother you. Fine, I personally command you to go hump like two sea otters right now! Go! *I understand that everybody isn't in a relationship nor am I condoning being a neighborhood tricycle where everyone gets a free ride! I am stressing the importance and benefits that come with sexual intercourse. If you do not have a significant other, try to find another outlet for releasing your pent up stress i.e. exercising more or joining a book club.

Psychology- Go see a shrink. Seriously, we are all crazy; it's just a matter of how much. Worst case scenario, it sucks - at least you get to relax on a couch and talk about yourself for an hour.

Injuries- Try a yoga or Tai Chia class. Learning how to control your mind is a long, hard process and these two classes will help. Be cautious of Bikram Yoga. I wouldn't necessarily put that in the relaxing category. It's in a hot-ass room performing Yoga and the instructors can sometimes be a little militant. As with anything, don't knock it until you have tried it. I'd suggest starting with basic beginners' yoga and then progress from there. Back, knee, and shoulder pain will slowly taper off as you become more flexible.

Nutrition- Visit your local farmer's market for fresh fruit and veggies. A lot of our meat and produce from the grocery stores are chemically altered shit – literally, GMO (genetically modified organisms). I'll tread lightly because these big corporations are assholes and are only concerned about their bottom line. Even store-bought honey is shit. The best food to eat is from your local farmers market.

Exercise- What is the single best type of exercise? Write every type you enjoy. Sounds corny, but it's the truth. You need to find that something special that makes you love to exercise. For some it's dance, others it's running. Find out whatever it is that keeps your happy parts happy and start doing it in juxtaposition with the VTD.

Chapter 2

EVOLUTION

Female ferrets can die if they don't mate. Once a female ferret goes in heat, she'll remain in heat until she finds a hump buddy. If she doesn't mate, her estrogen levels may become toxic resulting in death! HOLY SHIT!

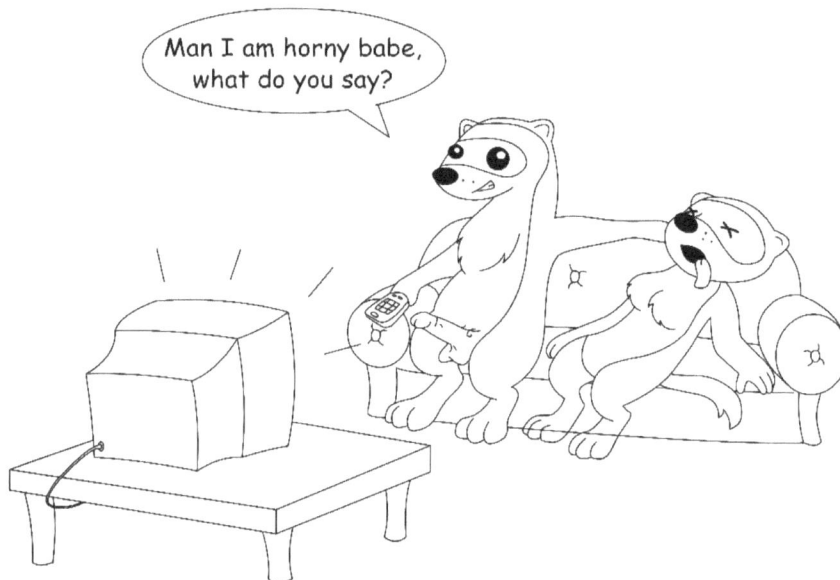

Evolution has produced some pretty amazing characteristics for human beings. We have evolved from little pieces of aerobic goo into land animals that can exercise, walk, breathe, talk, and have wild monkey sex via anaerobic pathways.

As horny cavemen, aka Neanderthals, our bodies were conditioned to flourish in times of plenty and conserve during meager periods. If there was not enough food, our autonomic nervous system would signal our metabolism to start slowing down. Luckily, we had fat reserves to keep us alive during scarcities – droughts, harsh winters, etc. When the days turned into weeks, the autonomic nervous system sounded a red alert, "warning, you are jeopardizing your fat reserves, you dip shit. It's time switch into conservation of fat mode and jettison muscle." (Yes, our autonomic nervous system uses cuss words and smart words like jettison.) This was an adaptive mechanism for survival. Muscle is a higher metabolic tissue than fat; it takes more calories to keep muscle alive than it does for fat. Muscles are like tiny babies, when they're hungry, they will tell you. If you don't feed them regularly, a piercing cry will sound to feed them, or else. In this particular instance, your muscles atrophy in order to conserve fat. This survival instinct was exactly what we needed as cavemen, not as humans today. I will cover wild monkey sex, big boobies, large penis', orgasms and the starvation state in chapter 5, so just keep reading.

Muscular Imbalances

Our sexy ancestral cave cousins passed on a lot more than the DNA that tells our bodies how to react during times of starvation. For one, just like the male heart, men have larger brains than females. Kidding! Many of my students believe me when I say that; it's pure comedy. Ok, our brains are the same size, but it's true with regards to the heart. The most apparent passage of our lineage can be seen in our musculature. The role of men and women as Neanderthals was black and white. Man wandered for miles in search of food. Women stayed at home, made clothes, tended to the children and prepared for the return of their men. Think about it for a minute and consider what those activities of daily living actually were? Men walked for miles until they came across a herd of animals; the hunting ritual would then commence. They would analyze the situation, take cover, and slowly approach for a kill. Once within striking distance (probably less than 100 yards), they would charge in an all-out sprint, jumping, and clawing their way until their prey was defeated or vice versa.

Females on the other hand, would be talking about Cavebook (the equivalent of Facebook), crafting goods and coaching pregnant moms about what to expect with motherhood. Muscle physiology and endocrinology (study of hormones) plays a huge role in how our genes have developed over the years. Why do you think the majority of men cannot touch their toes? It's from all of that jumping and sprinting which made our hamstrings stronger and overdeveloped. Or, it might have been rocks and shit that the wifey was throwing at us for checking out the topless neighbor; probably the former, but who really knows.

If we do not strengthen our quadriceps and stretch our hamstrings, we eventually create a muscular imbalance. Why do you think females have stronger quadriceps? Child bearing capabilities have developed the quadriceps to withstand an additional 20-30 lbs. from carrying a child. The overdeveloped quadriceps accompanied with a wider Q-angle (width of pelvic bone for birthing) makes women as much as five times more likely to injure a knee ligament (ACL aka anterior cruciate ligament) than males. Besides our genetic disposition, inactivity has also played a role in muscular imbalances. Take a look at the average desk jockey. Men and women are continually hunched over staring at a computer screen - this is referred to as Upper Cross Syndrome. This positioning is unnatural and creates weak upper and lower back musculature. Four out of five Americans have low back pain. Here is why. We sit too much and stare at porn all day!

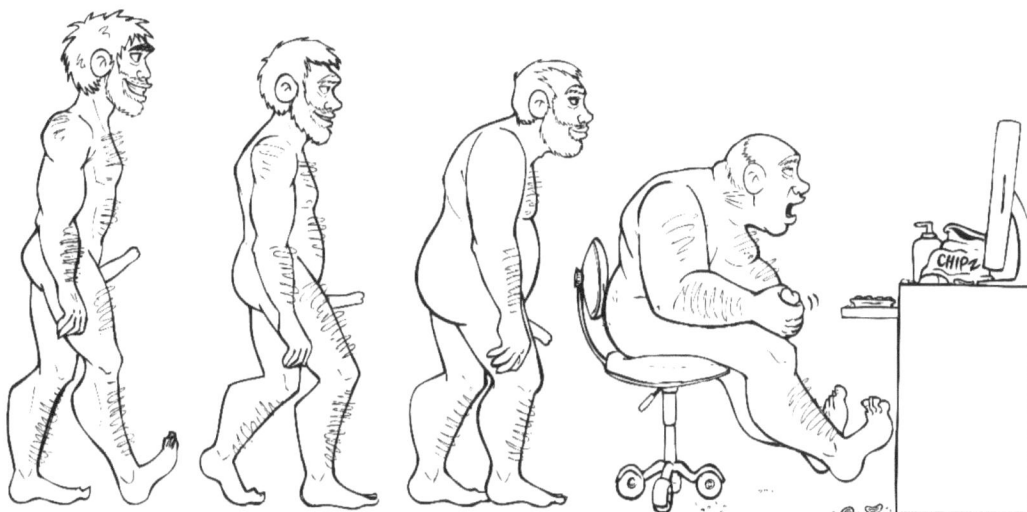

Ok, let me give you some muscle physiology real quick. One of the reasons we may have low back "pain" (which is usually associated with weakness) can be explained via our mechanics from a seated position. The hip flexors are long, powerful muscles that lie on the upper half of the leg. Their main action is to bring your knees to your chest as seen in sprinting. Today, sitting 7-10 hours a day causes them to shorten and pull on the pelvic bone (hip bone). It doesn't matter if you're looking at porn or instant messaging Becky from "It's Just Lunch" (dating site, get with the program!) your lower body is positioned in constant hip flexion. The opposite muscles (glutes) become inhibited and can't do their job aka glute amnesia – your ass forgets how to work! This unequal pulling mechanism results in an anterior pelvic tilt. The anterior tilt in turn shortens our erector spinae muscles (low back); beyond a neutral spine, which yields a constant pull aka pain. There are many other reasons for low back pain such as: too much belly fat, inactivity and weak upper back musculature. Constant repetition causes muscular imbalances and weaknesses in the body. I will teach you how to fix this via proper postural assessments, stretching, foam rolling exercises and strengthening the weaker muscles. (See chapter 4 for Injuries)

Hormones: Fight or flight (FoF) Response

Imagine the following scenario: It is a lucky day for you and the missus; you just got the green light from your cavehood friend that they would watch your kids for the day. You two horny toads scamper off into the wilderness to get your hump on and make some more babies. All of the sudden a saber tooth tiger jumps out of the bushes and you're now eye–to-eye with this beastie son-of-a-bitch. Your sympathetic nervous system kicks into gear and releases a shit ton of neurochemical reactions. The man that you are, you put yourself in front of your woman and tell her to run while you decide to fight (you FIGHT, she FLIGHTS). Your hypothalamus sends a message to your adrenal glands and, within seconds, she can run fast and get out of danger, yet, you can hit harder, see and hear better, think faster, and jump higher than you could only seconds earlier.

Cortisol, a catabolic hormone that breaks down fat for fuel, is immediately dumped into your blood stream. Your heart is jumping out of your chest two times its normal speed because of the important catecholamine (epinephrine aka adrenalin.) This hormone increases mental alertness and heart rate and dilates your arteries, sending nutrient-rich blood to the muscles. Within .15 seconds, you're officially ready to kick some tiger ass! Luckily for you, it wasn't a man eating tiger; just a super horny one who decides to have its way with you - better than being eaten alive!

All of these hormonal responses have been passed on. Even though we do not encounter the extreme situations as our ancestors did, we experience fight or flight (FoF) routinely (war is the exception). Studying for exams, traffic, presentations, fights with significant others, and even first dates trigger the exact hormonal responses. Every time your sympathetic nervous system triggers the FoF for situations that are non-life-threatening, you experience a false alarm. Too many false alarms and your body becomes exhausted. Constant stress without proper sleep, your body becomes exhausted. Working eight hour shifts without exercise, your body becomes exhausted. Eating shitty, nutrient-depleted foods, your body becomes exhausted. Pretty much everything in the American lifestyle triggers this response – we're fucked unless we address the S.P.I.N.E.™.

Mr. Cortisol (For more on Cortisol, see the Hormone Chapter.)

Cortisol is an amazing hormone which is produced by the adrenal glands (organs on top of the kidneys) to increase blood sugar levels – the adrenal cortex to be exact, but who's checking. Don't let me hear that shit, "Cortisol is a bad guy," because it's not. Without it, horrible endocrine diseases such as Addision's can develop and be life threatening.

In times of excess, cortisol gets its negative connotation by causing inflammation, weakened immune system, and muscle breakdown. It also damages brain cells in the hippocampus (part of the brain that deals with memory and is the first area affected during Alzheimer's disease). Through these stressed out times, we begin to place our body into an inflamed state. Literally, our blood and tissues become more acidic; consequently, increasing the likelihood for sickness, headaches, high blood pressure, sexual dysfunction, heart disease, and cancers.

Cancers thrive in acidic environments and that's exactly what you have done to your body during times of prolonged stress. Cancer is bad, don't get me wrong, but sexual dysfunction, now that's messed up! We are causing 80-90% of cancers because we are too stressed, inactive, and eat like shit! Our stressed out jobs and livelihood are creating stressors that are killing us. Even worse, it's affecting our hump time; What The Fuck! (Ironically, if I were to use the term WTF, it would be socially accepted – my dad still feels that it's inappropriate.) It's time we take a look at ourselves and ask if this is the life we really signed up for. A moment away from the glum and guess what helps reverse all of these horrific side effects of stress? Sleep, nutrition, exercise, and stress/behavioral management...S.P.I.N.E.™! You're not quite ready for this sucker yet, so keep your panties on, or take them off, whatever works.

Did Cavemen Cheat?
You bet your hairy butt cheeks cavemen cheated. I'm talking about cheat meals, not infidelity, because we all know that they were humping everything in sight! In today's diet market, we constantly hear fad words like "eating clean", "cheat meals", and "cheat days". Simply put, a cheat meal is eating whatever the hell you want. At Taco Bell, order four #3s! You're out for dinner: get a piece of cheesecake with your burger. The idea behind cheat meals didn't originate over the past few years, cavemen were doing the same thing. Unlike our fat asses, they were doing it for survival. Once a big mastodon was killed (a big ass hairy elephant with ivory tusks and gigantic cocks) they would gorge on it until they couldn't move. That was their cheat meal, but they were doing it for survival. The massive influx from fats and proteins open the flood gates for all sorts of hormones to pour into the body – cholecystokinin (CCK), Leptin, Ghrelin to name a few.

Insulin is released when we ingest carbohydrates - they were not in abundance back then, mainly just fruits and vegetables. Our bodies enjoyed this downpour of hormones every once in a while. As for today, it is the same – every once in a while. It keeps our system in check. Ironically, it's the exact opposite now. The majority of our meals are cheats: fast foods, vending machine snacks, sodas, and carrot cake muffin tops with pecans from Starbucks. These choices are man-made - low in nutrients and pretty much a perfect equation for explosive diarrhea! If we switch our eating behaviors around, cheat meals can actually be a part of our diets. Even though it is anecdotal evidence; consider my eating habits. I eat super clean Monday through Friday. I usually eat breakfast within 30 minutes of waking up. Some days I'll fast. I drink a gallon of water a day. Each meal consists of fat, protein, and carbs; my carbohydrates are solely from nuts, fruits, and vegetables. After my workouts, I consume the majority of my carbs to fuel my muscles for growth. I eat until I am 80 percent full - picture perfect! I am extremely disciplined because I know I eat whatever the fuck I please on the weekends: pizza, sandwiches, liquor, beer, wine, late night binges at Taco Bell, bottomless mimosas- you name it, I consume it. Guess what happens on Monday morning? Back to regulated eating and no binges until the weekend comes around again. The best part of my eating habits is that I have no cravings during the week. My body understands that it will get its free-for-all during the weekend. According to this, I eat 75 percent clean and workout intensely six times a week for 60-90 minutes. My default program is healthy. It's time to change your behavior around, and my diet plan does exactly that.

I may sound like a weekend drunk, but I'm just a fucking human being like you are. I indulge and have urges, but I put the work in and control my emotions so I am not self-conscious come summer time. Just imagine if I didn't drink, I would be on the front of every magazine cover Herculean style! Life without booze, hookers and drugs isn't my style. Actually, just the booze- but pretending to be a bad boy gets all the girls excited. I enjoy being a drunken idiot and having fun because life's too short to restrict ourselves to that extent. We need to find a happy medium. If you want to lose that spare tire, start by making mini sacrifices – prep your meals, drink water, eat breakfast, and take out the processed man-made foods. If you aspire to be that figure model, then eat 100 percent clean and eliminate alcohol – oh God, I just imagined that life. More importantly, remember, anything is possible - I will marry Lacey Chabert from Party of Five and you will get into the best shape of your life by adhering to the VTD.

We need to increase our activity and eat better – wow, I sound like a chick running for a Ms. American Pageant! It is true and that simple; eat sparingly and less processed. I'm not going to get all hippie on you and say you can't eat anything that is man-made- that's stupid and unrealistic. I don't want you to adopt an *Amylophobia* (fear of starch), but I believe that we should eat what's most natural and stay away from processed foods; chips, white breads, pastries and candies – I know, all the fun stuff! I will go into more depth on grains, but I believe a large portion of our diet revolves around grains, which we should restrict, and, better yet, time around working out (nutrient timing in chapter 5.) Is it a bad argument to say that grains make us fat? Every argument has two sides. People weren't fat when Jesus was breaking the bread with his disciples during the Last Supper. On the contrary, excess adiposity in JC's day was a sign of wealth - yep I'm erudite; told you Dad, I can use big words.

I have a lot of ideas about why we are fat, but I can't quite put my finger on it. Somewhere along our journey as *Homo sapiens*, something was lost in translation. Cavemen were not fat, it wasn't suitable. Not by caveman societal norms, but more Darwinian - survival of the fittest. If you were a fat ass, you would have been eaten. Evolution passed on the higher echelon of the gene pool- eliminating the slow, cowardly and pitiful (only if they would've eliminated the annoying). If you wanted to survive back in those days, you needed to be on top of your game daily. Times have changed - we are fat, lazy, and full of excuses. If we were attacked by man-eating tigers (not the gay ones), 66 percent of Americans would be taken out and eaten alive. The modern man works 40-plus hours a week, has a family and financial problems. He doesn't exercise, if at all, sleeps poorly and has sex three or four times a month, maybe – how pathetic! The more stressors that we experience (whatever they may be), our body senses these situations and we defend ourselves (physically, emotionally, and intellectually) as if we are encountering the saber tooth tiger again. Consequently, our adrenal glands are working overtime. They could become fatigued and/or fail to function. This is exactly how chronic illnesses sneak up on us.

Milo of Croton & the Principal of Overload

Some say the first documented example of resistance training came from a Greek man named Milo of Croton. Milo was a bad ass 6th century wrestler who was obsessed with cows. Probably not, but this is how I am going to tell the story. Did you ever question your grandpa when he told his WWII stories? I think not. So shut up and listen up to Grandpa Chris!

The story goes that Milo carried a baby calf every day to prepare for the Olympics. As you know, the Olympics are every four years; so as the time passed, the calf grew into a huge bull. The principal of overload states that progressive overloading will tax the human movement system (nervous, muscular, and skeletal system) by forcing it to become stronger and adapt. So, as the bull grew, the HMS was stressed, Milo adapted and got stronger. The citizens witnessed Milo blossom into a strapping young lad with broad shoulders, boulders for legs, a chiseled mid-section, and a huge cock!

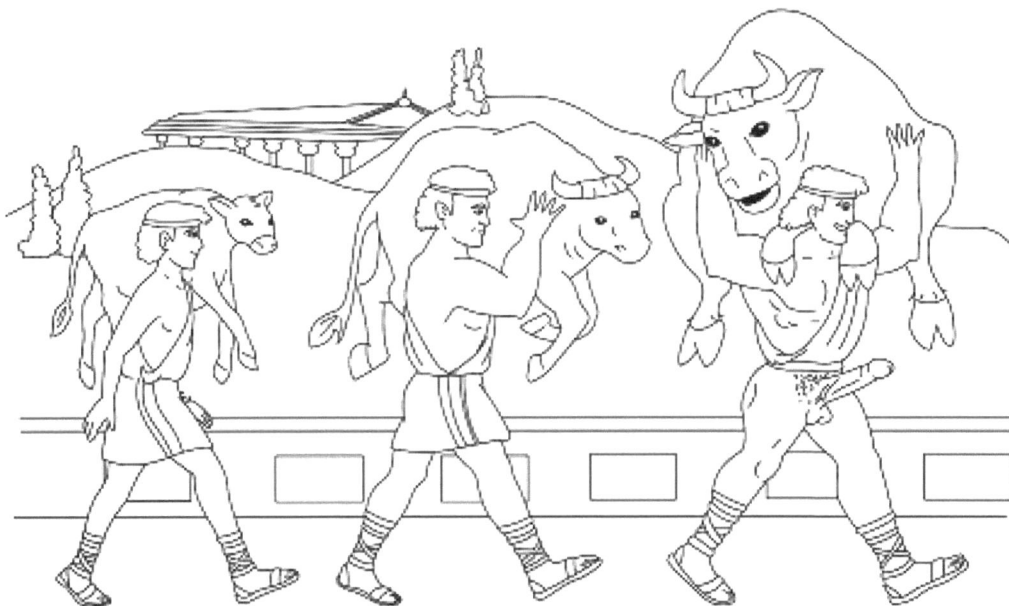

What did we learn from Milo? Continual repetition gets the job done. We need to adopt this basic principal while adding weight. Each set, more weight and work until you cannot push or pull anymore, aka volitional fatigue. This occurs when you can't lift another rep without cheating. It's important not to compromise weight for form, so maintain that good posture. If I could carry a big ass ox to work every day, his name would be Big Chief. Imagine when I would Show Up to work with Big Chief. All of my students would know that I am there for business; it's time to pay attention or else Big Chief's horns will be up your ass! Milo did not lift the bull once a week, it was every day. There was no shake weight, miracle drugs, electrical abdominal belts, or stupid ass 1200kcal diet plans to get him there; just tough hard work. We need to adopt this idea of progressive overload and exercising daily. It begins with movement. Begin with smaller goals. If you are sedentary, begin by exercising 2-3 days a week and progress into 5-6 days. VTD will teach you a proper progression that fits for everyone. Not too fast or restrictive- just perfect.

A lot of our fitness and nutritional failures come from setting the bar too high. Twenty grams of carbs for the first week! Fuck you. Many people will not be able to adhere to this and fall back to their unhealthy behaviors. It is important to have realistic goals. By following the VTD, the results will come together in a timely, realistic manner. This is going to be a nice long race people; it's called life. Ask yourself when were you in the best shape of your life? If the time frame is more than five years ago, then your journey is going to take a while (greater than six months). If you are expecting to lose 20 lbs. in a month, go chop your arm off, because it isn't going to happen properly. You may hit that magical number that you are aiming for, but in the end, you'll put it all back and probably even more. Weight loss is different than fat loss.

There are many factors that contribute to fat loss: clean nutrition, hormonal balance, controlling your stress, managing inflammation, adequate sleep, and a great sex life! I will cover it all and change your life once and for all. We live in a fantasy world and think that fat loss happens overnight. It's a process, ladies and gents that I will teach you. Now is the time to get on the VTD jet plane. If you decide to ignore my words and search for excuses or short cuts, you'll remain a tub of lard. As Michelle from *Full House* said, "How Rude!" You know what they say about nice guys? They finish last. But I go an extra step. They don't even finish the race, they are getting butt rammed by all the assholes in the world! Shut up and Show Up!

What happened to Pheidippides?
While I am educating you on all this exercise history, let me tell you the story of Pheidippides and the history of marathons (for the sake of butchering his name, we are going to refer to Pheidippides as Mr. Bare Ass).   Mr. Bare Ass was a hero of Ancient Greece. He was a herald who carried a message from Marathon to Athens that the Persians had been defeated. Upon his arrival (he was naked, hence Bare Ass), he gave word of victory to the kings and then immediately collapsed and died. The run was 26 miles. Folklore states that the lazy ass king of that time increased the total length of the legendary trek by .2 miles so that it could end at the king's gates. As of today, a marathon is a race that is 26.2 miles in length – tribute to Mr. Bare Ass!

Why the hell did I just ramble on about Mr. Bare Ass? It's to get your noggin thinking about what long duration cardio actually does to the human heart. The VTD isn't going to prescribe endless cardio because that recommendation is a shitty one. We were not designed to run 20 or so miles; we were designed to walk. Walking, not running, was the way of life as cave people. So why do we run and do so much cardio? People sure as hell don't run as a part of everyday activities - unless they are running from a bee, trying to catch a bus or sprinting out of the bedroom after a one night's stand. And that's about it. For one, when we do any sort of moderate, intensity exercise for longer than 90 minutes, we begin to break down muscle. This lowers our metabolism and gives the softer appearance. Just compare a sprinter to a marathon runner; enough said. Secondly, the amount of wear and tear on our ligaments and joints is extreme! A person has performed roughly 1,500 repetitions during a 1-mile run, just image 26 (carry the one, that's like 10 thousand reps, right?) Lastly, when we do steady-state exercise for extreme time periods (60-plus minutes) we begin to produce inflammatory markers that damage arterial walls. I have had two different students tell me that they knew people who have "mysteriously" passed away from running long distances. One was a teacher in his mid-40s who appeared to be extremely healthy, yet died in his sleep. Another student ran a marathon where someone died during the race.

Cardiologists are beginning to suggest that we could potentially be damaging our heart tissue during these extreme races (Dr. James O'Keefe has an awesome TED talk on it.) When we resistance train, microscopic tears happen on a cellular level. Well, it just could be that these same exact microscopic tears are happening inside our hearts. Now don't get all melodramatic on me and stop doing cardio, that's not the message of Mr. Bare Ass. If you're constantly running more than 120 to 140 miles a month, this message might be for you. It's the repetition that we are performing. Compare running a marathon to a car. The more we run, the miles on our car go up. The question is, how many miles will it take before your car stops working? If you're concerned, do your own research and talk with your physician.

How to fix your S.P.I.N.E.™?

Sex - Spice up your sex life by adding what I call the "fantasy box." No, it's not a magical vagina, get your mind out of the gutter. It's a box for each of you to put in fantasies that may be fulfilled (within reason, I'm not having a three-way with another dude, no way)! Agree upon terms and then every week take turns picking from the box. Yippee, naughty professor dress up! Oh fun, a new toy for cunnilingus! C'mon people, know your PC lingo for munching on box!

Psychology - Buy a large calendar. Post it up in the bathroom or somewhere in your house where you will constantly see it. Post progress pictures, motivational pictures and inspirational quotations (see chapter 7 for awesome quotes.) Write out your workouts and challenges. Visually seeing your goals on a daily basis will better your chances of success i.e.: 1. Eat a tomato a day. 2. Drink 10 glasses of water. 3. Smile more. 4. Eat more hair pie / slob more knob. 5. Bring Chris some Rock Hill Farms single barrel whiskey.

Injuries- Eighty percent of Americans have low back pain. By strengthening our core and glutes, we can begin fixing this problem. Start by doing a plank for 3 sets of 15 second holds for the core. For the glutes, start off with floor bridges for 3 sets of 15. As with any form of exercise, challenge yourself by changing the FITT principle Frequency, Intensity, Time and Type.

Nutrition- Invest in a wok. I use it to cook up a bundle of asparagus, head of cauliflower, two bell peppers, head of broccoli, one onion and one sweet potato - this lasts my fat ass only one to two days. I soak it with Braggs Liquid Amino Acids (less sodium), a boat load of Sriracha sauce, and 3-5 cloves of garlic. After 15-20 minutes you'll have enough veggies for at least half the work week.

Exercise- Look into a meet-up group. There is a website where people with similar goals can meet up and socialize, learn, relax, and/or exercise together! Meet ups are usually free, too.

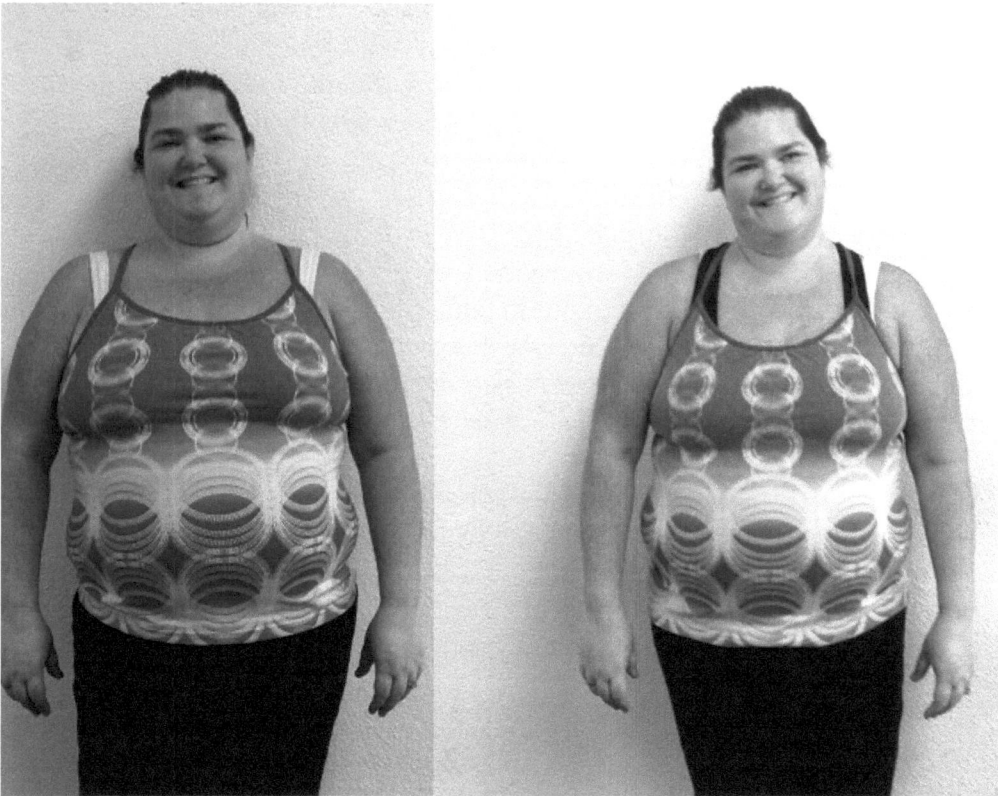

Client 1:

Beginning weight: 239lbs @ *46% body fat
Total S.P.I.N.E.™ score of 11

Results after 12 weeks:
227lbs @ *40% body fat (lost over 20lbs of fat)
Lost over 8 total inches
Total S.P.I.N.E.™ score of 20

Comments:
Diet: "I liked how I felt without all the grains and starches. The first two weeks were very difficult, but the energy levels that I had after were well worth it!"
Hardest workouts: "The hardest (but also most satisfying) was the superset of incline dumbbell press into dumbbell rows."
Favorite cheat: "Frozen yogurt after a hard workout. YUM!"
Biggest success story: "Throughout most of the program, I wasn't seeing the changes physically, but my friends were. My clothes fit me much better and some even fell off to the point where shopping was necessary. I have muscle where there was predominantly flab!! I am stronger and I feel healthier. My overall participation in this program has been a very positive experience."

* Body Fat Percentage education:
Essential body fat for women = 8-12% / men = 3-5% (needed for reproductive reasons and proper brain, heart, and physiological functioning.)
Average for women = 25-31% / men= 18-24%

Chapter 3

The Human Body

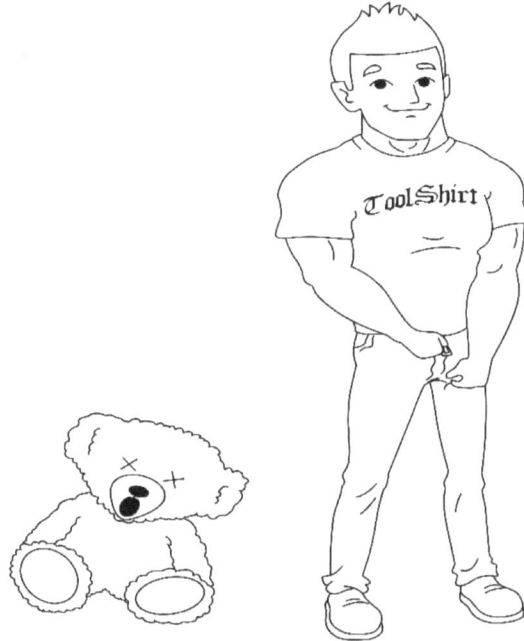

Did you know the human body has 206 bones? Sorry guys, we don't have 207 because of our boners - good joke, though! Muscles, on the other hand are a little more complex. Some anatomists believe certain muscles are connected while others believe they are separate - tomato, tomatoe. That total number is somewhere between 650 to just shy of 700 – that's quite a lot! There are even muscles that people lack. The Psoas minor (near the hip bone), for example, is only present in roughly 40-50% of the population. The Plantaris and Pyramidalis are small muscles of the knee and the pelvis region that are missing in 10-20% of the population. The body has many remarkably unique facets! Let's pretend for a second that I am as cool as *Bill Nye the Science Guy* and examine a few.

The pH (power of hydrogen) of our stomach can be as low as 2. For all you chemistry dropouts, pH is a number conveying the acidity (0-6.9) or alkalinity (7.1-14) of a solution on a logarithmic scale. To put it into perspective, battery acid is around 1 and citric acid (found in name brand sodas) is around 3. Acidic environments could break down some metals, bones, and your teeth enamel. The stomach secretes protective mucus via mucus membranes in the wall of the stomach. Luckily for us, that gooey shit prevents the stomach from digesting itself – pretty cool and disgusting at the same time! Another one is your epiglottis. This tiny piece of cartilage covers your esophagus (food pipe). When you swallow, a reflex triggers the epiglottis to cover the trachea (wind pipe) so food doesn't get into your lungs. Ever swallow too quickly and hear someone say "food went down the wrong pipe?" That's actually true. Food started to go down the trachea because your reflexes weren't quick enough. That's why you automatically hacked up a bunch of stuff all over your desk when you coughed. Lovely, I know, but that natural reflex just saved your life! Without the epiglottis, food would become trapped in the lungs, resulting in a bacterial infection and then probably death.

Ohhhh, you want more fun factoids? A man's refractory period (the time it takes for a man to cum again) can last between one minute and an hour. Guess what the largest determining factor is for the recovery time? Exercising and practicing a healthy lifestyle – HOLY SHIT! So, for you guys that want to start humping aka every man, gay or straight, start hitting the weights and stop ignoring her bean; that's where the magic happens!

ASS DOG

Ever wonder why men have fat bellies and women have chubby thighs? It's not that you are cursed from the fat Gods; it's primarily due to your genetics. The word ASS DOG is a kick-ass acronym for the main factors that affect a person's ability to adapt to exercise: Age, Sex, Specificity, Detraining, Overtraining and Genetics. When in doubt, refer to ASS DOG and you will probably find the answer.

The last two words of the acronym (detraining and overtraining) and the last "S" (specificity) relate to exercise. If you take a month off from working out, you'll return weaker and atrophy will set in (detraining). Overtraining happens when you work out three times a day for seven days a week without taking any rest days. Your body will begin to display signs of extreme fatigue, soreness, and you'll become weaker - a lot like the flu. Specificity is explicit to the type of goals that you want. If you want to run faster, sprint. For a bigger chest, do more push-ups. To develop a more functional body, increase power, speed, and agility via body weight and resistance training exercises. The most important factor determining your outcome depends on the type of exercises that you are performing.

Genetics is a huge factor that predicates a person's ability to adapt to resistance and cardio training. Do you think the Williams sisters, who are tennis stars, have an advantage over their female tennis opponents because of their stature? Hell yes they do! They are freaking yoked and can smash a tennis ball harder than most men can. Their musculature is attributed to an abundance of fast twitch muscle fibers, which allow them to perform movements faster; more on muscle fibers later. Did they buy these fibers at the store? No, it was passed on to them via their parents' awesome DNA. Albeit, hard work does pay off, but having a great deck of cards to begin with doesn't hurt the equation.

Android Vs Gynoid Obesity

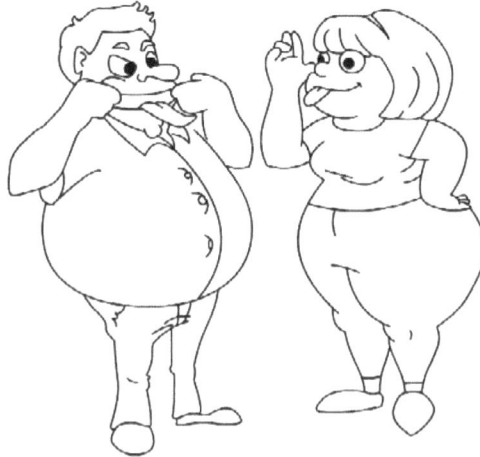

Apple: Excess belly fat Higher chances of heart attack

Pear: Excess butt and thigh fat

SPOT REDUCTION

These six factors are extremely important when analyzing one's goals. The problem with exercise is that people believe that you can exercise a problem area and "boom shake the room" - they'll be in better shape! Sorry folks, this is called spot reduction, and, to date, it hasn't been proven to be very effective. Our media has inundated us with information that suggests the possibility of reducing fat at certain areas. If you want a flat stomach and perfect thighs, then perform thousands of repetitions. It makes perfect sense to the lay person, if you want to lose fat around your thighs, arms or stomach, you should do a bunch of repetitions. Unfortunately, this is futile. The theory of spot reduction has people spending hours of time in the gym with zero results to show for it. Remember when you found out that there is no such thing as Santa Claus? Yeah I know: tears and cuss words. That is still the worst day of my life when my brothers told me... last year!

Fat and muscle are two different types of tissue. At no point in time can we turn fat into muscle. This is a common misconception that I hear trainers say on a regular basis. There are 3,500 calories in 1 pound of fat. If I want to burn a pound of fat, I need to put in the required amount of work. Crunches and leg abductions will not elevate my heart rate high enough to burn many calories. To burn a pound of fat, I need to incorporate larger muscles so my heart has to pump harder and faster. Guess what muscles those are? Guys, please don't say your penis because your penis isn't even a muscle. It's made up of cavernous bodies which are a type of tissue that allow for expansion. So shut up with the dick jokes. The answer lies in your legs along with other multi-jointed exercises such as push-ups and pull-ups; anything that mimics these exercises as well. To this day, the most overused pieces of equipment are cardio, ab, and thigh or glute machines. Sorry, ladies, you will not sculpt your body by spending hours on these machines. Rarely do you see people with awesome bodies running for hours, doing hip abduction machines, or hundreds of crunches - that's where the fat people are. The guys and girls in the best shape are the ones doing high intense exercises with heavy lifting - not the oh-so-pretty pink-colored ones. Defined legs are developed by performing multi-jointed exercises like squats, lunges, hip thrusters, push-ups, chin-ups and max jumps (the exercise chapter will clarify everything on multi-joints).

If your goal is to tone up your legs, train your legs every day (specificity)! If you desire toned and sexy arms you need to start doing push-ups and chin-ups every day. In regards to the midsection, we need to do more legs. What what what?!!! Yes, legs. Your legs are the body's largest untapped resource. Every person in the world has a 6-pack. It's a matter of whether we can see them or not. Our inner polar bear has been preparing for winter and has taken over by storing excess fat over our abdominal muscles. Guess what? Unless you live in Russia, it's not fucking winter, so start doing more legs!

To see our abdominal muscles, we need to lose fat, and, abdominal exercises do not expend many calories. By engaging our legs more, along with practicing proper nutrition, we will begin to see those sexy lines in our stomach. Have you ever heard of that saying "abs are made in the kitchen"? Well, they can be, but the secret truly lies in your legs. If you are not working your legs out 3-5 times a week, you're not working out properly. Put down this book right now and do 15 body weight squats into a chair! Seriously! I am not talking about a full leg workout, just a few sets per day; anytime you want to do abs, opt for a set of jumps, push-ups or lunges instead. I guarantee you'll flatten your tummy faster than performing all those idiotic ab exercises that you see personal trainers doing with their clients – yet their clients are still fat. Wow, I am a dick, but the truth hurts! Before you know it, you can share success stories like mine. I have saved a lot of money because I use my abdominals to wash my clothes. They are literally like washboards because I do legs four times a week. Dammit, that was a tool comment. Ok, tool comment number one has been documented.

MIRROR MUSCLES: MEN

I made that tool comment for a reason. One, is because it is funny and I know you laughed. Two, I can segue smoothly into the topic of mirror muscles. Girls are crazy and guys are idiots – it's unequivocal! Guys are typically very simplistic and animalistic in their ways (excluding myself)! We strut about, smacking our chest, trying to be the alpha males around females or other males. The belief that girls are attracted to sexy abs, nice arms, and a block-like chest keeps our pea-size brains occupied with barbaric behavior. Ladies, how many times have you complained when your man shakes out of his 7 For All Mankind® jeans only to expose his chicken legs? I know you have seen that toolish guy with huge biceps and rounded shoulders who constantly wears athletic pants to the gym. It is not impressive to be a lopsided penis puffer with a huge upper body and tiny lower half. In my opinion, it's pathetic. Guys, don't give me that genetic donkey shit either, because your legs want to grow. Our legs consist of 40% of our total body mass and should be our largest assets. Not only does it allow for growth in our lower AND upper body, but by engaging our legs more, we can burn more calories. Not sold? Well then try this Prince Albert on for size! Working your legs releases powerful hormones like testosterone and human growth hormone. The amount of work that must be performed to release the same amount of anabolic hormones via an arm workout is insane! Why workout harder, when you can workout smarter with better results? Another pet peeve is ignoring your glutes - you know, your ass, that thing you sit on. Are you afraid of being able to bounce a bowling ball off your derrière? To me that sounds pretty awesome! Your glutes are some of the body's most powerful muscles, so why aren't you working them out? FYI, leg presses should only be used on beginners, otherwise the machine sucks. Stacking five plates on each side doesn't do much for your glutes. There is limited hip extension therefore engaging them minimally. I like to compare the leg press machine to training wheels. In the beginning, they're needed and are a great segway into other exercises like: hack squats, Smith machine squats, deadlifts and lunges. When was the last time you saw a thirty year old riding his bike with training wheels? If I did, I would throw a fucking water balloon at them- no way! As with the presses, after a few weeks, you need to ditch them. Also, when you're done being a knuckle head, take the fucking weights off your machines; don't be that prick!

The bigger our lower half is, the larger the upper half can grow. How many guys want a 6-pack? If you do, then listen up. You need to start doing more legs. If you want nice abs, the answer lies in your legs. Bigger arms – workout your legs. Your legs are literally the Holy Grail. We become too focused on what we can only see in the mirror. Unlike our female counterparts, we only check out our front side when we narcissistically gawk at our bodies in the mirror. Therefore, all of the muscles that we cannot see are underdeveloped because we can't see them in the mirror. Our legs, back, and glutes are all left for the atrophy Gods - not to mention muscular imbalances. I can hear it already, "legs are too hard, so I'll just do calves." Stop it you pussy; learn how to squat, hip thrust and deadlift properly. The reasoning behind all this calf shenanigans is due to the attire we wear during summer – board shorts expose only our calves so we forget about our thighs – wow, we really are idiots! By neglecting the muscles that we can't see in the mirror, we set the human body up for failure and settle for mediocrity.

Let's take a closer look at our friend Sequoia Sempervirens - that's the scientific name for the Redwood Tree in Northern California (FYI, another spelling is Sequoyah and he was a famous Cherokee Indian Chief). How many towering Redwoods do you see with massive 30-foot branches yet have a small base? Very few; Mother Nature won't allow it because it would get blown over... TIIMMMMMMMMMBBBBBBBBBEEER! Have you ever said that word before? It's fun; say it next time you're at Starbucks and just wait for the reactions. The bottom line: the stronger our legs are, the greater potential our upper extremities have to grow and for the body to prosper.

MIRROR MUSCLES: WOMEN
Ladies, ladies and ladies, I have a love-hate relationship with your species. I love the way you walk around only wearing my extra-large Texas & Gonzaga t-shirts, but I hate how you perform endless cardio. I love your thoughtful actions, but I hate it when you lift 5-lbs and do bicep curls. I love the way you show off your cleavage, hate it when you spend 10 minutes using the abductor and adductor machines. Lastly, I love it when you perform sprints and lift maximal weights, hate it when you talk about periods. Seriously, come on. Anything that bleeds for seven days and doesn't die is considered…SPECIAL! Don't get your panties in a bundle, it's all in good fun, my species is just as SPECIAL. But, kudos when it comes to body recognition because you know your body like your husband knows the starting lineup for his favorite sports team.

You have an addiction to these exercises because you think they will "shape, sculpt and lift" – they won't. I believe in the following happy-medium: males should lift lighter weights with better form and females ought to lift heavier. No more crunches, hip adductor/abductor machines and/or 45 minutes on the elliptical. NO MORE, pipe it, CIERRA LA BOCA or in *Wedding Crashers* terms, "shut your mouth when you're talking to me!" I wish I could hire a ninja to stroll around gyms and throw ninja stars at those who use them. I wouldn't want to kill any of you, just small puncture wounds that would heal in a few days. I tried posting a link on Craigslist but my link was banned – Qué Cabrón (what a bastard)! Instead of focusing on your smaller muscles, let's focus on larger ones by doing more complex movements like the ones listed in the exercise chapter.

I understand the difficulty in hearing this message from a man so let my friend Christina take over for a second, "Hey girls, seriously, you want a sexy back, perky tits, awesome legs and an ass to die for, then listen to Chris. I have followed his programming for months and everything he said was true. I began by becoming comfortable lifting my body weight by doing tons of push-ups, bodyweight squats, lunges, floor bridges, and planks. I progressed into heavier weights, sprints, and lots of jumping and it was super spectacular – I looked amazing naked! The most important thing was being consistent and working out a minimum of five days a week. I now see curves I haven't seen since I was in high school! It really was that easy – I Showed Up and listened to what he had to say! Try it for a month and see for yourself!" Sorry, that was me again. I really did try to talk in a high and spunky voice, but seriously, do it. I can say this; the female and male students who have listened to my words 100% received their best body ever. All the girls in these pictures are students that I have taught or trained.

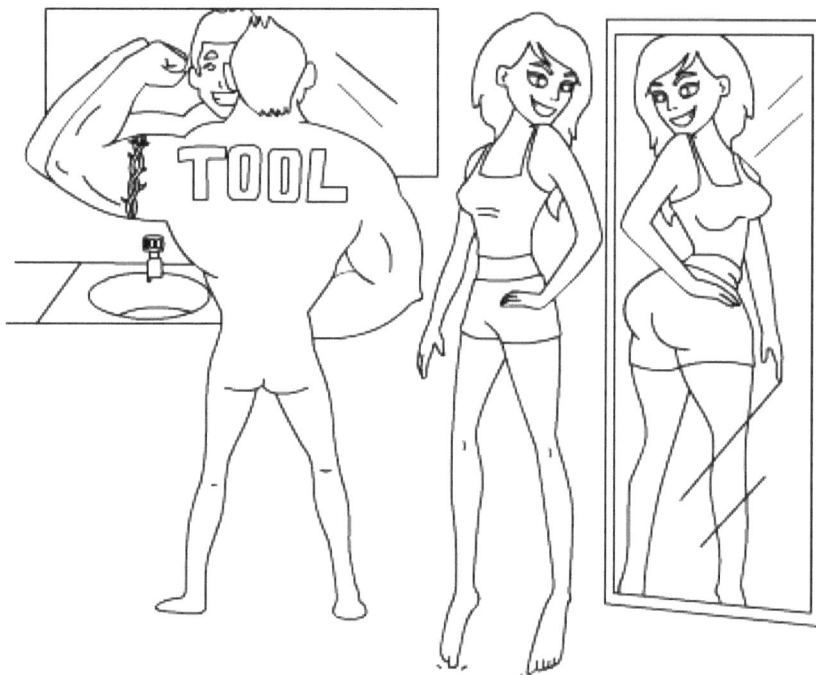

MUSCULAR IMBALANCES:
Another, and more serious problem with only working mirror muscles, is imbalances. Imagine the following upper body split routine: Day 1: chest. Day 2: back. Day 3: shoulder. Day 4: legs and core. Let's pretend that the person (let's call him Johnny Affliction) knows how to workout and he hit all three rep ranges: Strength (less than 6 reps), hypertrophy (6-12 reps) and endurance (12-20 reps). He is even educated enough to understand the rest periods and how it takes a minimum of 3 minutes during strength training to sufficiently replenish muscle glycogen. Let us take a look at Johnny Affliction's workout....

Day 1: Chest

Bench Press, 5 sets of 5

Dumbbell Incline Press, 4 sets of 8

Chest fly, 3 sets of 15

Day 2: Back

Cable Row, 5 sets of 5

Pull-ups, 4 sets of 8

Lat Pull-downs, 3 sets of 15

Day 3: Shoulders

Dumbbell Military Press, 5 sets of 5

Military Press, 4 sets of 8

Lateral Raises, 3 sets of 15

Day 4: Legs

Back Squats, 5 sets of 5

Front Squats, 4 sets of 8

Dead lift, 3 sets of 15

Plank holds, for 15 seconds x 5 sets

Day 5: Metabolic Functional Day

Broad Jumps, max jumps for 10

Push-ups, max

Pull-ups, max

Hand stand push-ups, max

Jumping Jacks 30 seconds

Repeat for 5 sets

PROS:

Johnny Affliction is aiming at hitting his muscles two times a week. He has cardio mixed in there to strengthen his heart. I love how he is doing planks and not isolating his abdominals. He is even doing Plyometrics and hitting his clavicle region of his pectoralis major – Holy rat shit, maybe Johny Afflication isn't a huge meat head tool!

CONS:

Not so fast, Johnny Affliction. Let the doctor (not really, but sounds cool) take a closer look at all those repetitions. 5x5 = 25, 8 x 4 = 32, 3 x15 = 45 add in 25 and 32 more. An acute triangle is a triangle with all three angles less than 90°, throw in the Pythagorean Theorem and the aggregate mean is roughly 14. HA! I may pretend to be smart, but math isn't my forte. Thank God for Google, you can just Google random shit and sound smart! The real number is more than 160 repetitions to 0*. Yes that's right, over 160 repetitions for the anterior deltoid with 0 for the posterior deltoid – that's not even taking into consideration the functional day with push-ups and handstand push-ups! See, having an understanding of the human body is empowering. Performing exercises such as bench press and push-ups recruit the anterior deltoid along with the chest and triceps. When doing a cable row, lat-pull-down and pull-up, the posterior deltoids are not engaged nearly enough to balance out the anterior workload. That's why people have a shoulder day, right? Little do people know that when performing a Military Press, the posterior deltoid is not engaged, only the anterior and medial part. The deltoid muscle is one muscle with three regions. If we continue to exercise only portions of the muscle, an imbalance will develop.
*Warning: anatomy nerdy stuff. There are seven main muscles that are engaged when you extend your humerus - the posterior deltoid is one of them. The latissimus dorsi, teres major and pectoralis major will be picking up the majority of the slack, leaving the posterior deltoid minimally engaged. The point I'm making is we need horizontal abduction/extension (as seen in a reverse fly or wide-grip row) to properly even out all of our pressing exercises.

ILS aka Invisible Lat Syndrome and a little SMR
Johnny Affliction is one of many guys in the world possessed with this horrible condition. Buff guys like Johnny toot their horn by telling everyone how "tough shit" they are because they can leg press 600lbs and halfway bench press 315lbs. I am more concerned at why the hell your shoulders are so internally rotated that it looks like you have an invisible T-Rex sitting on your shoulders singing the song "Who let the dogs out!" I seriously have no idea how guys think it's cool to have this upper body discrepancy which is ever so properly referred to as Upper Cross Syndrome. The likelihood of future shoulder problems is greater than your ego! The best advice I can give instead of continually making fun of your tan, flamboyant green shirt, and spiked hair is to stretch these tight muscles, strengthen your weaker ones, and properly apply foam rolling aka Self-Myofascial Release (SMR).

Fascia is a connective tissue that surrounds pretty much everything from muscles to nerves. I want you to imagine a bread roller; this will be your muscle. Now, stick the bread roller up your ass. Dammit, off topic, don't do that, sorry. I want you to imagine the bread roller surrounded with saran wrap. The wrap is a lot like fascia, it allows for surfaces to glide smoothly over another. Fascial highways can become tight or stuck together from inactivity, not stretching, previous injuries, and getting old – like tiny bread crumbs stuck between the roller and the wrap. If we don't address these affected areas, then arthrokinetic dysfunction will result from microscopic adhesions in the muscle. Let's use our brains and dissect arthrokinetic dysfunction. The prefix "arthro" we have heard before with arthritis, which means joints. The suffix "kinetic" means movement. Add in the word dysfunction and voilà, we have joints that don't move well. Think of the body like a chain link. The more kinks we have in it, the greater the chances will be for pain and altered movement patterns. Most guys don't stretch, but when we do, it's usually too late. Knots begin to formulate in the muscles and we try to undo a knot in the muscle by pulling on it as hard as we can (stretching). Ever try getting a rope unknotted by pulling on it harder? The inner caveman attitude takes over in order to fix the problem, "Me strong, me fix by pull harder," yet we only exacerbate the issue. The fix is foam rolling. I don't care if you think you look like a wailing pussy flap – foam rolling works wonders! Your current divergence is far worse than what others think of you rolling around on this cylinder. There are many different colors which designate the density of the foam roller. White, blue and any mixture thereof, are specific for beginners and pain-sensitive individuals. For the moderate peeps with a higher pain tolerance, there are black foam rollers. For the badasses out there, I personally suggest Trigger Point rollers, grids or PVC pipes. Some extremists will use wooden rods and/or barbells. This shit works too, it's just not for everyone. Understandably, you need to walk before you can run so for beginners, start with the white- or blue-colored foam rollers and then progress intelligently. Stereotypically, your chest, lats, calves, hip flexors, adductors, and upper traps are extremely tight, so we need to release this tension via rolling.

Guys:

Practice being able to touch your toes and touching your hands behind your back. Wake up every morning and spend 3 minutes stretching. Thirty seconds of jumping jacks. 15 seconds of rotating your arms and then torso. After the quick warm up, perform 2-3 sets of 15-30 second hold for each hamstring, followed immediately by touching each arm behind your head. I want you to do this twice a day. Shoot for another session at work or when you get home. Everyone has 3 minutes to spend; so Show Up and Shut up!

Girls:

Start off every morning with 4 sets of 15 reps of body weight squats, lunges, step-ups by using a chair, push-ups, and hip thrusters. I highly recommend using weights, but I understand the uncertainty for now. Take-home message for both sexes: unleash the inner beast and start working your legs out a bare minimum three times per week. If you don't, then settle for subpar with your clothes off... Show Up or Shut UP!

How to fix your S.P.I.N.E.™?

Sex- Try a new sex position. Missionary = boring! We have been doing that one forever. Try something new and exhilarating like the gladiator, reverse cowgirl, the butterfly or my favorite, Shake N' Bake! Not fucking with you either, it's an actual position. To do it, the man pulls out and puts the tip of his dick on the clit. Then, hold the base of the one eyed trouser snake and shake it as fast as you can from side to side so that the head hits the clitoris with every vibration. Shake N' Bake, baby! A great under $10 investment is a sex calendar book with a new and exciting position every day. Relationships die when the sex life takes a U-turn into the shitter - don't let it happen.

Psychology- Stare at yourself in the mirror for five minutes without saying a word. Mentally, I want you to say to yourself "I am a winner, I can do this. I fucking rock." Repeat this for five whole minutes. After you do this, you will have an extra pep in your step for the remainder of the day. Continue to do this until you don't need the mirror. You'll wake up every morning and know that you're sexy and the world is yours to rock!

Injuries- Steam Room. Not only will this help with relaxation, but it will detox your system, cleanse your skin and great place to work on flexibility. I go into the steam room for five to 15 minutes per day. I say a little prayer and then stretch by touching my toes, fingers behind my back, calves, inner thigh and calf stretch. My flexibility has never been better and I credit it all to the steam! Sex note...Awesome spot to try and sneak in a quickie. Two hot bodies rubbing up against each other with the sweat glistening and a chance of getting caught...BOING!

Nutrition- Prep your meals ahead of time. Choose two days in the week and spend one hour cooking. I enjoy watching a TV show that I recorded on the DVR while I cook up some chicken and veggies. I'll keep up with the market while I BBQ a prime rib. Who says you can't kill two birds with one stone, because I'm pretty sure I do all the time! Strive for one new dish a week. By turning into a student of the culinary arts you'll not only attract members of the opposite sex, but you'll keep your eating habits new and exciting!

Exercise- Wake up 45 minutes early and do the following routine three times: step ups on a chair (10 per leg), max push-ups (don't compromise form; remember one good push-up is better than five shitty ones.) Ten body weight squats and a plank. This should take you 15 minutes. Now, go walk, bike, or run for the remainder 30 minutes.

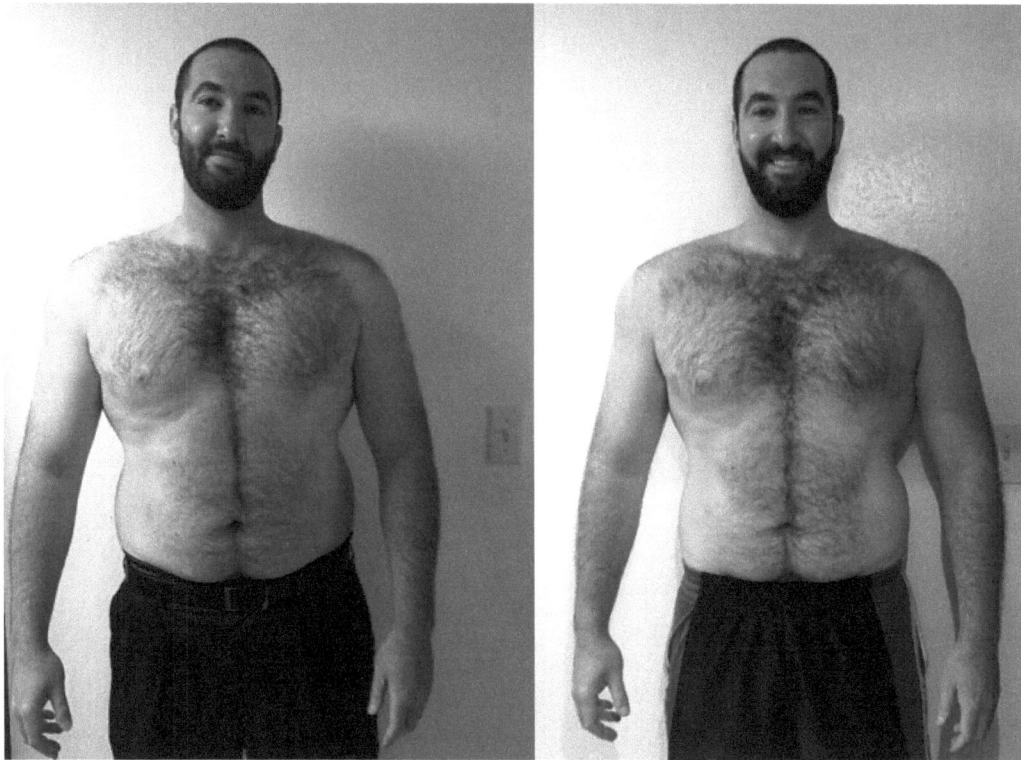

Client 2:

Beginning weight: 258lbs @ 25% body fat
Total S.P.I.N.E.™ score of 13

Results after 12 weeks:
247lbs @ 19% body fat (lost 17lbs of fat and gained over 7lbs of muscle)
Lost over 9 total inches
Total S.P.I.N.E.™ score after 23

Comments:
Workouts: "I enjoyed the variation week to week which kept things interesting and creative. Enjoyed learning new workouts and can't wait for more!"
Diet: "I finally understood what full is and how much (or little) food will satisfy. I enjoyed cooking more and meal prepping. Most of all, the money saved on eating in vs. eating out."
Hardest workouts: "The hardest (but also most satisfying) was the superset of incline dumbbell press into dumbbell rows."
Favorite cheat: "Sandwiches' after my workouts for nutrient timing!"
Biggest success story: "I decided to partake in the VTD challenge to try and get into the best possible shape for my wedding in four months. I adhered to Chris' diet and workout schedule as much as possible and thanks to him, I was able to feel great for my big day!"

Chapter 4

S.P.I.N.E.™: Sex/Sleep/Stress. Psychology & Injuries

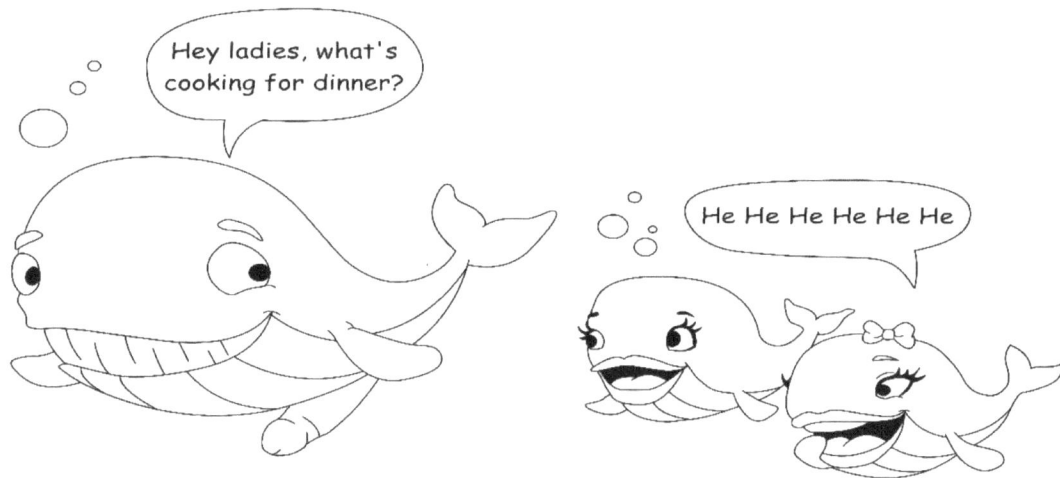

Hey ladies, what's cooking for dinner?

He He He He He He

"Yes! That's awesome! You just took a dart to the jugular" – Stiffler's role as the zoo herder in *Old School*.
"Wait, Wait, pull what out?" – Will Ferrell
"The dart man, you have a fucking dart in your neck" – Stiffler
"Ha ha ha, YOU'RE CRAZY MAN! I like you, but you're crazy man." Ferrell

Great movie, with plenty of nudity; *Old School* is a classic! This scene when Will Ferrell shoots himself in the neck with a tranquilizer dart is how I am going to start off this chapter. The average American has a five-inch dart sticking out of their neck and has no idea it's even there. The dart symbolizes not only how dysfunctional the average person is, but also how chubby wubby we are! We think everything is all dandy with our big bellies aka BBQ (big belly queen as my brothers say), spare tires, and fat asses hanging out. We try to walk a few days a week, order nonfat lattes and drink diet soda in an attempt to mitigate our escalating problem.

S.P.I.N.E.™

S.P.I.N.E.™ should really be SSS.P.I.N.E., but that wouldn't be as catchy now would it? The three S's stand for stress, sleep and sex. Psychology and injuries follow with nutrition and exercise ending it off.

Today, many people segment health and wellness into two categories: Nutrition and Exercise. It's like wellness is a big clown bicycle and if one of the wheels is flat we are fucked. Well, that sounds all fun and dandy, but there's more to it than that. "Diet is 80% of health and the other 20% is exercise." Go fuck a goat, no it isn't. Please explain this to a past client of mine who was working out five days a week and ate flawlessly. Why wasn't she losing any weight? Could it be because she was sleeping only four to five hours a night? Possibly. Or maybe it was the fact that she was freaking out that her "internal clock" was running out - she wanted to have kids by the time she was 35, and she was 35! Her "bicycle wheel" was functioning perfectly, but her S.P.I.N.E.™ was fucked!

What about a male client who trained with me four times a week, yet was gaining weight from consuming only 1500 kcals per day? Could it have been the divorce he was going through? Once again, his "bicycle wheel" was functioning perfectly, but his S.P.I.N.E.™ was fucked!

We need to look at a whole lot more than exercise and nutrition. I am going to dissect these seven aspects of health and wellness to give you a better understanding of how crippled our society is. If we don't start taking action immediately, then the 500 billion dollars that we directly and indirectly spent in 2010 on coronary artery disease is going to be pennies on the dollar! As you could tell from the nifty bold letters from this chapter, I will be focusing on S-P-I in this chapter and then proceeding with nutrition and exercise.

Show Up or Shut Up!

OK Chris, enough lambasting! Help us, what can we do? That's my specialty, helping others. That's why I decided to make pennies teaching (big thanks to all you teachers out there, you're fucking awesome!) In my opinion there are two things that you can do: Show Up and correct your S.P.I.N.E.™. One is easy and the other takes hard work. The first part is Showing Up.

I was sitting down one day venting to my brothers about how bothersome some of my clients were. We were discussing names for my potential company and Advanced Personal Trainers just didn't get the job done. After my vent session they looked at me and said, "Sounds like all your clients need to do is Show Up!" Bingo! It hit me in the face like a pair of awesome titties; out of nowhere - Show Up Fitness was born. I started to realize that all of my clients, who saw me at least three times a week and followed my dieting advice, achieved fantastic results. Others, who bitched about lack of time, had excuses for everything or just didn't want to change their habits, remained the same.

This was the beginning of my formula for S.P.I.N.E.™. I found out that showing up was a huge component. Additionally, mental state, stress levels, sex life, happiness, nutrition and injuries all played a role as well. How could I motivate and persuade my clients and students that the media was full of elephantitis, and losing ten pounds in ten days wasn't very likely? This was the motivation behind the development of my questionnaire which you will take in a second. Relax, as Toby Keith said, "I want to talk about me, I want to talk about I..."

Any trainer that tells you he/she loves all of her clients is lying. We go through rough patches just like every other profession. I've heard it all: loneliness, frustration, hatred, wives cheating on their husbands, and, vice versa! Sometimes it's an hour-long vent session! Maybe I should call myself Dr. Christopher Loren? At the same time, I have seen miraculous metamorphoses: overweight housewives transformed into MILFs, men with dick-e-doos (a belly that sticks out further than their dick does) who are now proud to take their shirts off and show off their new, defined abdominals, sub-par athletes who got cut the previous three years and then made the sports team, and clients with chronic pain who were able to reduce and manage it via exercise. I've trained many clients and the ones who listened and followed exactly what I said, achieved the best results.

No diet or workout program can be regarded as the number one way to lose fat - you should understand that! But, if you've tried diet after diet and program after program, it's time to listen to a professional and stop trying to take the easy way out. I have lectured for hours to students on what many professionals, myself included, agree are the best ways to lose fat; however, these three conditions are exemplified:

Client 1: Johny Jackoff.
Johny wanted what many guys want, i.e., lose fat and gain muscle. He ran five times a week and when he lifted weights, he did a ton of arms, calves, and abs. Many guys do idiotic workouts similar to this. If you think guys have difficulties listening or being sensitive in the bedroom, think again; the gym environment is way worse!

On top of his amazingly awesome workout schedule, he was eating like a high school girl getting ready for prom. He didn't know how to handle stress and complained all the time that he wasn't getting results. I instructed him to back off the cardio, rest, eat healthier, try meditation or some type of yoga to mitigate his stress, and give it at least a month. Two months into the class he quit because he didn't achieve the results that I promised. Before he pouted and left, I asked him what his workouts had been like. He told me that he kept on running, tried yoga one time, was afraid of eating too much fat because he would get fat, and was still doing a ton of ab and calf work. Johny Jackoff didn't listen to a single fucking thing I said. He did the same shit that he was doing before and got what he deserved: a spare tire!

Client 2: Susan Doveface.
Susan was a cute lady in her 30s and if she could lose 20-30 lbs she would be smoking hot! The ideal situation for this scenario would be a 3-4 month time span. She wanted to lose 15-20 lbs in a month for a friend's wedding.   She told me that she already ordered her dress three sizes smaller! I really wanted to say, "What the fuck!"   This was the first time I heard about this common fad that some girls take on.

Amazed by her optimism, I accepted her circumstance with delight, but told her it would be very challenging. Optimism is key here people. I never take on a client under false pretenses. There are people who have lost 25 lbs in a month through diligence and adherence to a program. I had a client for this book lose on average 20lbs of fat per month. It's possible, but realistically, 4-5 lbs was what I expected and anything more would be awesome! If you recall the movie, *Willy Wonka and the Chocolate Factory*, Violet Beauregarde didn't listen to Mr. Wonka. That little hussy went off and ate the gum even though he suggested otherwise. Susan was the same way. She snubbed my explanation and pushed toward her first session. I implemented five days of resistance training, caloric restriction, and 30-60 minutes of cardio either fasted or after her workouts. *In these unique *situations, proceed with caution due to overtraining and/or putting the body into a starvation state. Sleep and low stress levels will also be huge for success.*

As the month progressed, she would skip her cardio sessions and every weekend she drank in excess at least one night. I didn't expect anything less when she texted me that she couldn't fit into her bridesmaids dress. She expected amazing results by pussy wolfing around and not preparing for the battle ahead. If she would have set realistic goals and came to me a few more months earlier, we could have gradually introduced her into harder workouts and less calories. She wanted extreme results, so extreme measures had to be taken. So is life.

Client 3: Buttwad Brother Nick.

Ohh Nicky Boy. Never thought I would be writing about you in a book, did you?! Love you to death, but you're a bit of a poltroon when it comes to listening (he likes to use big words). Whether if it's the fact you don't want to listen to your younger stud of a brother or you're just a dipshit, I am not quite sure. Nick has been the same size since his early 20s (now mid-30s) and has always wanted to attain that six-pack and bulky look. Don't get me wrong, Nick's in great shape. He has a solid four-pack and fairly broad shoulders, but doesn't listen worth a monkey's cooter! He consistently does arms and abs, sometimes as for long as two hours. His neck and lower back hurt from the lack of leg and corrective work. I have told him numerous times to implement these strategies into his programming. He asks me all the time, "what are good exercises for the abs?" My response, "squats, lunges, chin ups and presses", yet he spends the first 30 minutes of every workout with his dumbass ab routine. He listens to the news, websites and random people on BART (Bay Area Rapid Transit) over his brother. I give it five years before his head falls off because he pulls so damn hard on his neck when he does bicycle kicks.

In the end, if each of the clients would have listened from the get go, they would have attained their results. Twenty pounds in one month? Yes, I am that confident in my abilities with that specific situation. Cocky? No. Concocky; it's the happy medium between cocky and confident - I thoroughly enjoy making up words.

Here are the main things to adhere to with the S.P.I.N.E.™ principle:

1. Train your large muscles first. You should begin with your legs, chest, and back before doing exercises for your arms or core. Large muscles induce a higher heart rate response and release more fat-burning hormones.
2. Multi-jointed exercises before single-jointed i.e. squats before leg curls, bench press before triceps, and pull-ups before abs. In juxtaposition with number one, the more joints that are working, that means more muscles are engaged, therefore burning more calories.
3. Stop wasting your time doing extended periods of cardio. Twenty to thirty minutes after your workout is awesome. Twenty to thirty minutes of HIIT is even better! Thirty minutes of steady-state running was big when Jane Fanda was shaking her fine ass in the 80s – not anymore! They say the best exercise is one that you enjoy. So if you like to run, be smart about it. Do a small weight training circuit before your run for 10-15 minutes to maximize muscle glycogen depletion (see chapter 6 for workouts.)
4. Stay the fuck away from the ab area. Spot reduction is like Y2K, a huge cock burger! It can't happen and more than likely will never be proven so. The idea is to rid the area you're working from the flab – it ain't gonna happen! I literally just counted some tool at the gym performing more than 100 crunches. He has probably had his gut for years and will continue to do so until he changes his stupid habits. Seriously though, the guy was wearing cologne,

dancing to his music, sporting a golden fake tan, and a cutoff shirt reading, "Who's your daddy." If I had one wish, it would be to point at people like that and have them disappear to dip shit island- ahhh the world would be a better place!

5. Be leery of grains. Grains don't make us fat, wink wink, (just so the big grain corporations don't ram an ear of corn up my ass and sue me.) If you're an athlete and want to eat grains, have at it. Your body can utilize the excess fuel and store for later use. Oh shit, I forgot that everyone thinks they're an athlete, so let me clarify. If you are currently training for a big event like a 10k, triathlon or performing more than two hours of aerobic exercise per day, grains may be for you. If that isn't you (which it probably isn't) then make sure to replace grains with more fruit, vegetables, and water!

6. Stop fucking stressing. Stress is like a rocking chair, it may be fun for a little while, but at the end of the day, you haven't moved an inch. Take classes, read books, listen to music, and learn how to breathe. If you don't learn how to relax and get a firm grasp on your stress levels, your body will not allow you to change. Sleep is one of the best ways to restore an overworked body, so make sure to offset your hectic life with plenty of it. High stress levels and a lack of sleep is like trying to study with a rock band playing in your room - fat loss is not gonna happen! During the VTD, you will learn how to condition your mind and leave your stressors at the front door.

7. Be happier. Sorry to be the bearer of bad news, but you're dying. So is everyone else around you. You have two options: bitch, moan, and complain about how that isn't fair, or, give life 100% of what you have to offer. I guarantee if you smile more, the world will be a better place. Oh ya, have more sex too. Sex is awesome, I am getting horny right now thinking about it!

Rude, touchy, and insensitive are a few words that may come to your mind. Sticks and stones may break my bones, but words will never hurt me (FYI, my thumbs were totally in my ears and my tongue was sticking out when I wrote that.) I've heard it all: prick, asshole, loquacious, hung like a blue whale, and my favorite, thunder cunt (sounds like a super hero right?) Whatever your angle is; I don't give a rat's ass! Our nation isn't listening. We need a hard slap across the face along with a swift kick to the groin. There could be a TV alert, "Caution Caution Caution, Americans, you're fat and killing yourselves." Irascible Americans would try to fast forward the station or change it to some stupid reality TV show. I'd suggest something funny like *Duck Dynasty,* so you don't have to hear vacuous girls whining! Those girls are about as worthless as condoms- I prefer the pullout and pray method! We know the statistics, 30% of Americans are obese and, in 2030, we are projected to be even fatter, topping the charts at 42%! Granted, these charts are based off the Body Mass Index (BMI), which is a guesstimation of adiposity and does not considering muscle. People bitch all day long and say the BMI is hogwash, but it's quick, efficient, and the last time I walked downtown, I sure as hell didn't see many in shape people. We're fat, let's face it. Let me help teach you how to fix your problems with ideas I have put many hours into formulating. From my working experience with doctors, nutritionists, psychologists, and physical therapists, I created the acronym S.P.I.N.E.™ which I believe is the answer to our fat waistlines and costly health problems. There will always be aberrations, but for the most part, if you listen to the VTD and try your damnedest at correcting your S.P.I.N.E.™, you will achieve whatever your heart desires.

The S.P.I.N.E.™ Questionnaire

Stress, Psychology and Injuries (SPI) = 33%

Question 1: Do you sleep between 8-10 hours a night? Y=1

Question 2: Do you stretch or foam roll at least 3 times a week for 15 minutes? Y=1

Question 3: Do you spend at least 1 hour per week disconnecting from societies fast pace way of life (praying, going to church, meditating, something spiritual, walking by yourself, reading a book, painting, massage, yoga, or tai-chi)? Y=1

Question 4: Do you have a negative outlook or are you a Debby Downer? N=1

Question 5: Do you smoke (cigs, tobacco, and marijuana)? N=1

Question 6: Do you have a hangover two times per month or drink more than 3 drinks per night? N=1

Question 7: Are you easily frustrated or get angry like the Hulk? N=1

Question 8: Are you a worry wart or constantly feel rushed? N=1

Question 9: Do you have low back pain or easily injured? N=1

Question 10: Do you have sex at least 3 times per week (with yourself doesn't count)? Y=1

Total S.P.I.N.E.™ Score:

Nutrition = 33%

Question 11: Are you currently on a diet or have tried one in the past three months and stopped? N=1

Question 12: Do you have cravings for sweet or salty foods more than 1 time per week? N=1

Question 13: Do you eat at least 10 servings of fruits and vegetables per day? Y=1

Question 14: Do you eat breakfast? Y=1

Question 15: Do you eat more than 2 meals per day (including snacks)? Y=1

Question 16: Do you drink a minimum of 8-10 glasses of water? Y=1

Question 17: Do you eat fast food more than 4 times a month? N=1

Question 18: Do you drink soda (examples include: Diet, vitamin water, Gatorade & energy drinks)? N=1

Question 19: Do you eat cereal, bread, tortillas, rice, or chips more than twice per week? N=1

Question 20: Do you have a designated cheat day or meal per week? Y=1

Total S.P.I.N.E.™ Score:

Exercise = 33%

Question 21: Do you exercise 4 days a week (min of 1 hour per session)? Y=1

Question 22: Does cardio make up more than 50% of your exercise (walk, running, biking etc)? N=1

Question 23: Do you spend more than 15 minutes per week isolating your ABS (TOTAL)? N=1

Question 24: Can you perform 10 regular push-ups (girls, off your knees) 20 regular (guys)? Y=1

Question 25: Can you do 1 chin-up (females) 2 pull-ups (males)? Y=1

Question 26: Do machines, body weight exercises or DVD's make up more than 50% of your exercise program? N=1

Question 27: Do you perform resistance training 3 days a week (min of 45 min per session)? Y=1

Question 28: Do you watch more than one hour of TV per day or you sit more than six hours a day? N=1

Question 29: Can you touch both of your hands behind your back AND can you touch your fingers to your toes? Y=1

Question 30: Do you use resistance on your legs more than twice per week? Y=1

Total S.P.I.N.E.™ Score:

How to Read It.
The human spine has three distinct curves: cervical (upper), thoracic (middle), and lumbar (lower). There are 33 bones incorporated, counting the sacrum and coccyx regions. The regions work together to allow for proper movement and support for the rest of the body. If one of these regions becomes displaced forward (kyphosis) or in the lumbar region (lordosis), pain throughout the rest of the body can occur. Have you ever tweaked your neck and then have had pain in your arm or chest? Sciatica is caused from the compression of either the lumbar or sacral nerves which can have radiating pain down your entire leg. When the S.P.I.N.E.™ is jacked up, the rest of the body suffers.

The same goes with S.P.I.N.E.™. If one of your groups of ten questions was below 7 (70%) then you need to fix it. As in school, 70% is a pass- that's what you're aiming for. The average score for my clients was 4.5 per section. I had a few people with a total score less than 10... TOTAL. What does that mean? That there are a ton of improvements to be made and they're going to see the best results with complete adherence. If you scored well in S-P-I and E, follow my nutrition plan to fix the N portion and the rest will adjust itself. A common complaint I hear is that "I've tried everything." There is this impenetrable "5-10lbs of stubborn fat" that will not disappear for the life of them. After answering these questions, we discover that there is more to the equation than the original five-pound fat loss goal. After we sit down and make a realistic program, fat loss happens.

Patience is a virtue; I tell everyone to give it a solid month before they notice a change. It is important to note that when there are levels of high stress, lack of sleep, inactivity, and poor nutrition, the likelihood of change is low. This metabolic tornado puts the body into a poor scenario for fat loss. The perfect example was a client whom I trained three times per week and she worked out three additional days on her own. She worked 50+ hours a week, ate like shit, slept only a few hours a night and despised her husband. Her monthly check-ins were constantly disappointing even though I prepared her for them. Weight gain was inevitable because her S.P.I.N.E.™ was poorly balanced. Even though her score on the E portion was moderately high, overall, she was a train wreck (she received a S.P.I.N.E.™ total of 12). Eventually, she was able to lose fat, but that was after a two-month hormonal intervention with a doctor. Remember, exercise is a stressor, so if you're highly stressed and begin a high intensity training program, you may be doing more harm than good!

The amalgamation of these 30 S.P.I.N.E.™ questions came from interviewing many clients, students, and professionals in the field. As with anything, I am sure it could be better, but I think they best encompass the pillars of wellness. Make sure to read each question thoroughly because it's not as simple as it looks. The reason I didn't word each question so that all "yeses" receive one point is because I want you to really think about what it's asking. The end goal of these questions isn't to achieve a perfect 30, it's to track your successes and see the improvements. When you begin to fix your S.P.I.N.E.™ score, you'll notice fat loss, muscle gain, increased energy levels and improved self-confidence.

The highest score I have ever seen was 28 (thank you.) My back is tweaked and when I drink, I turn into a gremlin and scream for Taco Bell; I swear that's why I don't have hangovers. I need to thank my sexy girlfriend (LBI) for putting up with my midnight rants and morning farts - they can be bad! There may be some questions that make it impossible to get a high score i.e. sitting more than four hours. That's ok. That question was built to add awareness. Do your best to move around every couple hours. I challenge clients to do push-ups every hour. I am not talking hundreds, whatever you're capable of. When you energize your physical being, all of a sudden your mental state improves and productivity increases.

There are some questions that may raise the hair on your back: 3, 20 and 22. I believe the S-P-I portion of the questionnaire is arguably the most important aspect of S.P.I.N.E.™. If you're highly stressed and not resetting your system via sleep, plain and simple, you're fucked! Allowing yourself to enjoy a nice hike, take a meditation class (yoga, Tai Chi), getting your nails done (no phone), sun bathing or reading for an hour all help you to detach and reset your dials back to homeostasis. Some sort of detachment is needed to reestablish your natural settings. If you're constantly driving in first gear, your body will eventually overheat (see stick shift analogy under stress!) Look at your agenda and take the time to schedule in some "ME" time. I am not asking you to find time, I'm telling you. It's something that needs to be done for your sanity. Life is way too short to constantly feel rushed, ease off VTDers!

Do you really need a cheat meal? No. Do Americans have self-control? No. The all or nothing mentality works for a select few. If there are no cheats or some sort of leeway for the masses when it comes to diets, the likelihood for success goes down the shitter. I personally don't call it a cheat meal. I know when I have put in the right amount of hard work and have adhered to my diet system long enough that having a piece of cheesecake won't set me back. The key ingredient is self-control, which takes time to condition. I consistently see people begin a restricted diet plan and within two to three weeks sabotage everything because they couldn't handle it. They indulged in some "do not eat foods" and feel like it's the equivalent of cheating on their spouse, so they implement the See Food Diet: Ben and Jerry's, pizza, pasta, you name it, if it's in sight, they'll eat it! It comes down this, we are humans with real life events. In the next three months, you will encounter birthdays, weddings, vacations, holidays and special events. It doesn't mean you have to be that food Nazi who stares at people in disgust because they are eating a slice of bread. Here's my trick: workout the morning of the event (ideally, fasted) and save your calories for the evening. When it comes time for that event, I turn into a pig, literally! Food will be hanging from my beard while I scoop out the next food victim - its feast or famine, baby! I indulge because I know there won't be any setbacks. I have more muscle than the average person. My metabolism is higher and the extra calories will be used to build muscle. And, I love free shit! The next morning, I'll wake up and workout twice as hard. The moral of the story isn't to be like me. It's to understand self-control. Own your decisions and don't fall privy to emotional eating.

The last question that may raise some eyebrows is #22 "does cardio make up more than 50% of your exercise?" Cardio has numerous health effects, but a program that consists primarily of cardio can potentially place your body into a highly stressed and catabolic state. Again, these questions were developed to add awareness and implement weight training. Running places an abnormally high amount of stress on your skeletal system. It doesn't strengthen your bones nearly enough to prevent osteoporosis and the lack of hip extension inhibits gluteal development, aka your ass becomes weak without proper resistance training. If you like running, have at it. But I'll bet you 18

Rocky Mountain Oysters that if you take a month off and replace it with weight training, your body will feel and look, better. As always, the best exercise is the type that you love. If signing up for a 10k or half marathon is your fuel to start exercising, that's awesome! I just want your body to remain intact!

Many people praise cardio over weight training. Well, I say to each his own. Cardio will minimally increase your metabolism and not strengthen bones insofar as weight training does. Cardio is great, and it helps decrease the chances for coronary heart disease (CAD) and that's why I have you do it at the end of your workouts. As a total percentage, it's about 20% of the workout program. Weights will yield a stronger, superior body than cardio. What type of body would you rather have? Soft and skinny or strong and defined?

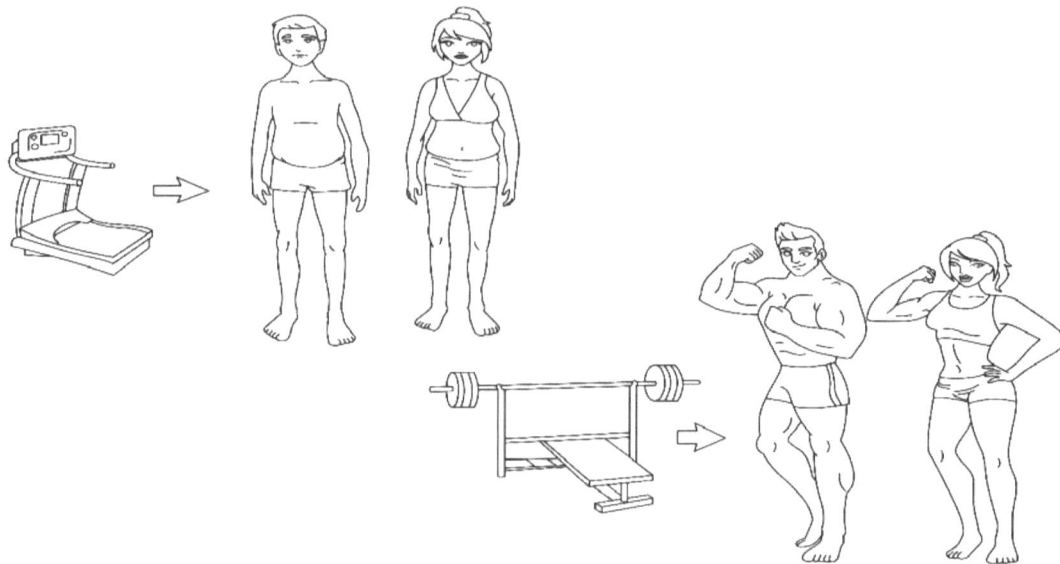

Cardio makes you "Skinny Fat"   *Weight lifting makes you Strong and Sexy!*

Additionally, if you score poorly on the following questions, I suggest visiting your physician for a physical to see if any other intervention is needed before beginning. In the end, I want your success, but it needs to be attained in a safe manner.

1. Sleep less than five hours per night?
2. Smoke or drink regularly?
3. Currently going through a divorce or extremely unhappy with relationship status?
4. Under extreme stress at work (constant deadlines, checking email/texts constantly/worried about getting fired)?
5. Has something extreme happened within the past three months? Family member has been hospitalized, lost a job, had a child, divorce, been diagnosed with a disease?

S.P.I.N.E.™: Stress

We need to stop playing the pity game and realize that everyone has stress. I bet you 25 pig testicles that I can find someone with higher levels of stress than you. We're built to handle stress in small amounts and it's actually beneficial. The human body is like a manual car aka stick-shift for you non-car junkies like myself. When driving in first gear and inching toward the red line (RPMs are getting too high), we're supposed to push the clutch in and switch to another gear. This allows the engine not to work as hard. Constant stress is the equivalent of driving in first gear all day long - even on the freeway! If you don't allow your body to de-stress, the engine will blow a gasket aka heart attack. On top of everything, when you park the car in the garage at night (go to bed), you leave it idling high. This constant stress can lead to hypercortisolism (too much cortisol.) Cortisol is supposed to be at its lowest in the PM and highest in the AM, but when you constantly stress, you pull a switcharooskie. Lack of sleep due to high amounts of stress places the body into an exposed state of higher cortisol levels. Gamma amino butyric acid (GABA) is a neurotransmitter in the brain that primarily regulates neuronal excitability aka it calms us down. Hypercortisolism depletes GABA, which can be a reason why it's hard to sleep during times of high stress. The hippocampus aka "emotional brain" (looks like a fucking sea horse), is a part of the limbic system, which deals with emotions. In Alzheimer's disease, the first part of the brain to be affected is this region. Hippocampus atrophy, as seen in Cushing's syndrome, and PTSD (especially Vietnam), is becoming more apparent due to the extreme levels of cortisol. Essentially, the body becomes metabolically broken from overstressing and it needs intervention ASAP. You have compromised sleep, mood, metabolism, and energy levels in lieu of the American Dream. If you don't learn how to ameliorate stress levels, you'll continue to write the perfect equation for a heart attack, cancer, and a ticket to have grizzly sex with the Grim Reaper.

My Crisis

In 2006, I entered cooperate America as a client manager for one of the nation's largest banks. I trained a high up banking manager who offered me the job because of my ability to build relationships. The money was great, but the lifestyle sucked a wildebeest's asshole. I found myself drinking a pot of coffee a day, stressing regularly over deadlines and consistently binge drinking after work. I was still exercising, but only 2-3 times a week. There were more than 100 people on my floor and fewer than ten exercised regularly. One of the biggest shockers that I found was how many bankers smoked. Daily, I would see the same 15 – 20 people go outside for a smoking break. The moment I knew it was time to make a change was when I couldn't fit into a pair of my jeans - I was a fat ass! It took roughly two years of that crappy lifestyle for me to understand what I was doing to my health, and it took a solid four months to turn my poor lifestyle around, but I did it. Look at your lifestyle and S.P.I.N.E.™ score to see how long you have been treating your body like shit. Maybe you want to reconsider your time frame and make some realistic goals.

Americans have been driving in first gear for long enough and suffering from the consequences long enough. It's time to make a change and the VTD is the answer. Ready for the ball-breaking revolutionary pointers for alleviating stress? Exercising, eating more fruits and veggies, drinking more water, doing the naked dance, avoiding inflammatory foods (sugar, grains, alcohol, vegetable oils, processed foods and dairy), and more sleep!

S.P.I.N.E.™: Sleep

"I'll sleep when I'm dead!" No shit, Samuel Elliott, but lack of sleep is at the top of the list of what can bring you closer to six feet under. Somniphobia is the fear of sleep and that definitely isn't me, no sir! I aim for at least seven hours per night and try to get eight to nine during the weekend. A new baby typically results in six months of sleep loss for parents during the first 1-2 years of its life. Fucking kids, they make us fat, grow grey hair and miss out on sleep! As with creditors, debt can be a huge problem when it comes to sleep. Losing out on six months of sleep is huge. You can help manage stress by sleeping at least eight hours per night. The importance of this S in S.P.I.N.E.™ is the most important, hands down. Without it, you're worthless!

Chronic sleep deprivation will increase your chances for heart disease, high blood pressure, diabetes, stroke, and obesity. While we're on the topic, some seals and whales fall half asleep aka unihemispheric. Their brain hemispheres take turns sleeping, so they can continue surfacing to breathe; now that's a cool factoid! Another interesting one, Leonardo da Vinci was known for his polyphasic sleeping habits (taking quick naps instead of one longer one aka monophasic). Granted, his genius is unparalleled by any human, but he did die when he was in his sixties. Could that be due to the weird sleeping habits? Who knows, but it seems like today people are constantly trying to "body hack" and find short cuts, such as the poylphasic sleeping cycles. If it works for you, so be it, but don't start passing along the adage that less sleep is better, because that is definitely not the case.

A lack of sleep makes us age quicker and decreases anabolic activity. Sleep is required for cellular restoration and regeneration in the human body. During sleep, we release large amounts of growth hormone. This hormone is a huge player in cellular reproduction and when we begin to miss out on sleep, the body doesn't recover properly.

Sleep is a metabolic regulator; it's the Spyware for our desktop. Without proper sleep it's like surfing the web for hot Asian MILFS or girl-on-girl porn - Virus time! So you either download that spyware aka 7-8 hours of sleep or that porn is going to fuck you - literally!

The same happens during finals week in college. You get all hyped up on caffeine, stay up late, stress more, and sleep less. The result? A weekend cold or sickness because your immunity has been compromised. What happens if sleeping eight hours a night isn't in the equation? Try everything in your will power to make it be. If you can't, schedule in time for some power naps because they will save your life, literally. If you're a shift worker or someone who sleeps less than six hours, understand that fat loss will be extremely difficult. Unarguably, bodies are different. If you go to bed and restfully wake up with only six to seven hours of sleep, then you're maybe all right. I want you to truly understand what natural energy is before you start disregarding sleep as unimportant. Just because you wake up and grab a cup of Joe and all of a sudden have energy doesn't mean you received enough sleep the previous night. That's fake energy. Try to go a day without caffeine and see how your body responds in the morning with six to seven hours of sleep. I'd be willing to bet one double-edged golden dildo that you will be exhausted during the day. They say that when you get into your Teenage Mutant Ninja Turtle pajamas and go to bed, if you fall asleep within five minutes, you're sleep deprived. Bottom line: Don't fuck around with sleep.

Things to avoid: Exercising three to four hours before bed. You'll be wired from the release of the fight or flight hormones, but also you won't be able to sleep due to the increase in body temperature. Avoid excessive alcohol, bright lights, and caffeine after noon and definitely not past 5 p.m. The half-life of caffeine is between 4 and 6 hours. This means that it takes roughly that period of time for your liver to remove it from your body. If you are one of those annoying people (meaning I am jealous) who can drink coffee before bed and/or unaffected from caffeine, go fuck a jackrabbit you lucky SOB!

Helpful Pointers for Better Sleep: Read before bed. Try relaxation tapes. 3-4 ounces of red wine. WARNING TO ALL OF YOU DRUNKS! Make sure to measure it out. If you drink too much and get a blood alcohol content, your REM sleep will be compromised. To all you hot cougars out there, that glass of wine you just poured is not even close to one serving. Bullshit. The average pour at home is closer to 2 to 3 servings, which would be more than 200 calories! I'm not saying don't drink, just be cautious. Ear plugs work for me and for the light sleepers. Limit your exposure to television, cell phones, computers, and whatever the newest technology is that has bright lights. Warm milk may help. Not a warm glass of shut-the-hell-up *Happy Gilmore*, just your basic 2% milk. There are some who believe in taking a warm shower immediately before bed. Set the thermostat between 60-65 degrees or keep a window open. The cooler temperature promotes a decrease in core body temperature, which initiates sleepiness. You can try the mineral supplement Magnessium citrate. Magnesium is required for the proper functioning of muscle and nerves and can help the body relax before bed. Melatonin is the sleep hormone produced by the pineal gland during darkness. Be aware that some complain of crazy shit happening in their dreams. It would be one thing if it were awesome kinky dreams of sex, but, no. I'm talking about a midget unicorn who has a dildo as a horn and is beating you at a game of Candy Land. Weird stuff, so be cautious. This leads me into my favorite topic and best recommendation; sex. Doing the magical naked dance before bed and climaxing releases the chemical oxytocin, which helps promote a restful sleep. If you don't have a partner, then go beat the one-eyed trouser snake. Ladies, go plant some root. Find some pictures of whoever gets your funny parts engorged with blood and go have fun with it! What a perfect segway into the last S of the S.P.I.N.E.™.

S.P.I.N.E.™: Sex
Sex, everyone wants to talk about it and just about everyone is thinking about it. During coitus and/or climax (see I can be PC), there is a release of endorphins into the body. Endorphins have a similar chemical structure to opioids (like morphine.) Now, not to be PC, when we cum, the flood gates open with the release of endorphins which delivers an analgesic effect to the rest of the body (hence the want for a cigarette, and night night time for us guys.) Endorphins are involved in controlling the body's response to stress, regulating contractions of the intestinal wall, and temperament. That's why some of us fart and others need to go take a big poo-poo, but most of us are just super happy! So why aren't we humping more?
The top three reasons people are not having sex are: I'm exhausted, I'm just not in the mood, and I have a headache. Never thought I would be giving advice on sex, but here it goes. While I'm at it, my goal is to see if I can get you aroused during this next section, tell me if it works!

Excuse #1: I'm too tired. Great, then exercise! Exercise boosts circulation, shapes up the body, and primes the brain for sexual satisfaction. Vasodilation (increase blood flow) has a lot of positive sexual reactions: improved arousal, lubrication, genital sensation, and that little tingle in your eye as well as your penis and clitoris that says "Wow, I am super horny" - sounds good to me! The increase in exercise will not only produce more testosterone, but hinder cortisol levels (remember T is anti-catabolic) and improve your grumpy ass feelings through endorphins. We have all come across that grumpy man or woman with a stick up his or her ass who we want to say, "Go get laid already!" Unfortunately, we can't because the Human Resources Lady has tied our hands behind our back- I set you up perfectly, just use your imaginations and have fun with that one!

Ladies, ever get annoyed with your man when he pokes you in the morning with his nocturnal penile tumescence? Well, stop freaking out! Men produce maximal levels of testosterone in the morning, hence the unscientific name "morning wood." Take advantage of this situation and save a horse and ride a cowboy!

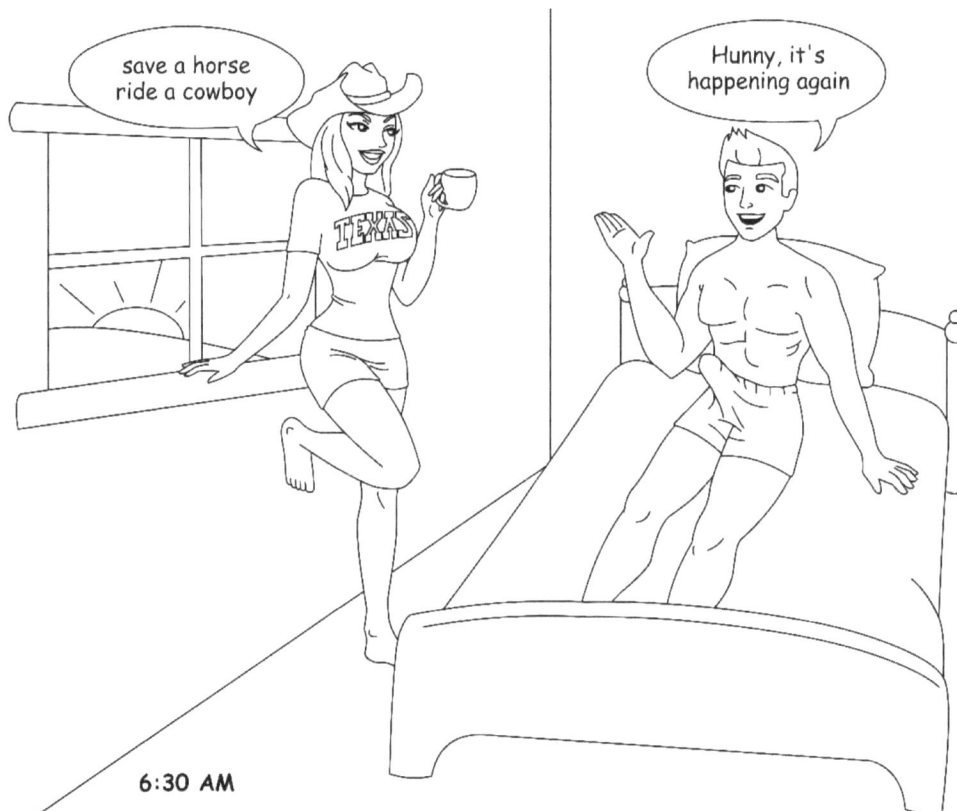

Instead of thinking of it as "quickie" think of it as barter! "Ok honey, we can play poke a kitten only if I get a 15-minute massage tonight after the kids go to bed." As a man, we are very sporadic and spur of the moment. Propositioned with that scenario, the vast majority of guys will take it in a heartbeat because we aren't thinking with our cerebrums! I've declined sex two times in my life. One was from a behemoth of a lady who I swore was a man and I didn't want to find out. Granted, I was sober. If you were to give me a few drinks, eight shots and another few beers, I would have definitely been game – that would have probably been one of the best nights of my life! I bet she would have made an amazing breakfast the next morning. She definitely hadn't skipped any of them. The other time, I was legitimately tired. I had a long ass day dealing with stupid grumpy people; as my brother Steve always says "Not feeling it!" The girl at the time was a square, but was feeling a little frisky. I gave her the ass treatment (not putting anything in the ass) but moreso, turning my ass to her, letting her know I was too tired. Looking back on that scenario, I wish one of two things would have happened. One, an earthquake struck and a beam fell on her head - that hooker stole money from me! The other, being she take the initiative to rile me up. With my newest lady friend, I found it doesn't take much to get Sasquatch up and ready to have some fun (that's an awesome name for a dick FYI!) All she did was start massaging, teasing my man area, and being extremely sexy and seductive in her ways. After a few minutes, I wasn't tired anymore - I was crazy horny! That was the best 38 seconds I had in a long time! Seriously, though, during the day, my boners don't go down! Sometimes I have to tuck them in during the day because they are sneaky sons of bitches and poke up out of nowhere!

For the average person, sexy time will not happen until the end of the day, so it takes some work - that's why it's called a relationship! Guys if your girl is tired, she won't respond very well to kissing her super-fast, while trying to take her bra off. Don't you dare use that line, "wanna fuck?" You might as well try throwing your poop at her because that probably would work better! That's about as sexy to women as it is for a man to hear his woman talk about her menstrual flow being heavy this month. Fuck that, it's not cute and doesn't work. If you're horny, take it as a challenge to get your lover horny. Give a massage. Kiss her sensual spots (neck, ear, bottom lip, belly button, CLITORIS). Send her some flowers or hide cute note cards in her purse. Drive to her work and place a love letter on her window. Cook her dinner out of nowhere. If you want to do the no pants dance, take action and make it happen! As a man, there should never be a time when your tutz (we need to bring this word for a lady back) isn't in the mood; make her! If you haven't discovered, Dick talk rarely works. You need to be her knight and shining armor. What ever happened to wooing your gal? Be creative and most importantly, have fun with it. Before you know it, she'll be begging you to pull her hair and man handle her in a fun, yet frisky and new way. Women love spontaneity and excitement, so grab those tiny testicles of yours and make it happen. FYI, girls, everything I just said goes for you, too, aka reciprocity!

Excuse #2: Not in the mood. The whole mood issue probably means you two sex pots need some spice and creativity. Try different things like toys or new positions- use your imagination and bring back that excitement from when you first met! Remember when you two were bonking daily? That needs to happen again. Bring back that magical fire and excitement. I call it sexual periodization. FYI, I am pretty sure you can throw any word in front of periodization and it makes you sound smart. Mammalian periodization! Electronic periodization, "Oh wow, he must be smart!" You just need to change it up before it gets boring. If you hit a plateau and don't address it, eyes start wondering. For the men its secretaries, nurses, and friends. For women, its bosses, pool boys, and friends. Fix it before it's too late. Find out what her fantasy is. My favorite is to make a sex box. You both put 3-4 things into a box that you want to do and each week you pick. Make it a date night. Go to dinner. Treat her like a lady; open her car door and hold all doors for her, you moron. Get a little tipsy and then explore those sexy bodies; it might be a good idea to have a mercy word such as "ARMADILLO PUSSY."

Excuse #3: I've got a headache. If your girl has a headache suggest more water; Americans are chronically dehydrated. If she doesn't like that nerdy retort, then try the same moves from the "exhausted state" but throw in some chauvinism. That's why cowboys rock. They haven't forgotten how to treat a lady. Guys today are huge pussies. They think too much with their small brain, which just gets you in trouble. If you're horny, use your brain on top of your head and ask to get her some aspirin or just start giving her a massage. A random act of kindness will put her in a better mood. If that doesn't work, try some red wine; nothing that a little liquor won't help. Worst case; tell her to go kick rocks! If those pieces of advice didn't work, your sex partner is a stress case and a square, so move on. Life is too short to find excuses. What if you were to get hit by drunk driver or struck by lightning, then what? You went to heaven without having sex that day. That's fucking insanely stupid and now I am upset! Shut up with the excuses and find time, because you won't

43

have any time when you're dead. Sex should be exhilarant, explorative, and pleasurable for both of you. As a couple, you should be striving for a minimum of four times a week; that's two times during the week and two on weekend. That's not counting oral either, gotta find some time for that, too! Make a sex schedule, get into porn or role playing; there is an answer to your hackneyed ways. Funny embarrassing moment about Chris. My mom once overheard my brothers and I talking about sex and duration. I was telling my story about this one time when I was with a Playmate (not even close, but it makes for a better story) and we were fooling around. I don't know what it is with you girls and teasing, but she was playing the hotdog-in-a-bun game. Grinding her ass cheeks around my enormously large boner. I am usually a boob guy, but after about 15 minutes of that jackhammering-ass-shit, before we even started having sex, I blew it, literally! From the kitchen I hear, "Christopher, are you a quick draw?" You can only hear my voice screech out, "MOM!"

Some helpful pointers: Eat better, drink more water, sleep more, exercise hard, and be more creative with a large dash of spontaneity. These things will help increase energy levels and testosterone production. Every girl I have been with gets crazy horny after a mid-day workout. Must be the sweat glistening off my rock hard body. Dammit, tool comment number two. But something during that workout jars something loose and brings out the barbaric side in one another. We literally go home and ravage one another. It's fun and exhilarating! Ripping clothes off, mounting her up against the wall as we stagger down the hallway. Passionate kisses - it's super-hot. I can only imagine what the neighbors think, "Oh that Chris, he sure loves his Animal Planet."

Holy rat shit, did you just see what I just did? Recommending exercise literally helps with everything! If you truly think you have a low sex drive, try getting your testosterone checked out.

S.P.I.N.E.™: **Psychology: Time to Show Up or Shut Up**
We all know what the road blocks are that stop people from changing: time, social surroundings (TV, friends), family, and significant others. Those excuses will always be there. One of my best success stories for this book came from a guy who just had a kid. He lost more than 42 lbs of scale weight - crazy fucking awesome! He could have had plenty of excuses why he wasn't able to perform the workouts or eat healthy, but he chose not to bitch. He used his brain and figured out times he could workout. He sacrificed sleep on some nights to wake up early and exercise. Communication with his girlfriend and family members was used to help babysit his beautiful baby daughter. That's how it's done folks, no excuses, just hard work and Showing Up!

We all have those demons that tell us to eat that piece of pie, go out for drinks, or persuade us not to work out. It's these choices that you make that will eventually define who you are. No one will ever put a gun to your head and say, "You better order that fucking Big Mac or else." No. It's a choice that you're making. I understand that you're hungry or you may have a craving. Does your brain control your emotions and body or do you control it? At the end of the day, you're the one who made the decision and you have to live with it. We make the same choices at Show Up Fitness, but we choose our battles and hold ourselves accountable for our actions. If we eat something off our plan, no biggie, we will make it up in the gym. Our default eating and exercise patterns are healthy, so we don't have to worry. The biggest thing to understand is that you are in control.

I hear bitching 24/7. "I can't study because of this", "my life is so stressed out", "I have so much on my plate" and "this is too hard." Ever seen *Dumb and Dumber*? Remember the scene where Jim Carrey is waiting for his "date" at the bar and a lady pulls up a chair and starts talking to him about her day? He slams his head into the bar and exhaustively yells "I DON'T CARE!" Well, enter that scene right here. There might as well be a template for excuses:

Dear "enter name of person you are about to bitch too",
Blah blah blah blah I'm so stressed out. Blah blah blah personal sob story. Blah blah blah poor me. Blah blah blah blah I am a pussy, please feel sorry for me. Blah blah.

Thanks for understanding.
Sincerely,
Pathetic.

Americans are turning into a bunch of pussies. We act like five-year-olds who get pushed down. We look around for someone to cry to and pamper us. What would you do if some Taliban dipshit came up and tried to take you? You're going to get tortured and probably beheaded. Are you going to roll over and pee on yourself? As Dylan Thomas best said, "Do not go gentle into that good night." Well put, D-bomb! You will poke eyes, bite, yell, and give 110% of everything that you have. Those penis puffers need to know that they fucked with the wrong person. Now ask yourself this. When was the last time you gave exercise and diet the same amount of effort? Tough love? You're damn right! I can coddle you and tell you how special you are, but at the end of the day, it comes down to the decisions you make when presented with those demons. What are you going to do? Show Up or continue down Pity Lane for the rest of your life? It's time to take responsibility for your actions and stop pretending that we're all Job from the Bible – Oh shit, I just made a biblical reference! Yikes, and I just cussed. Blasphemy? No, God and I are cool like that.

In talking with friends, students, and clients who've all made health related changes, I found a consistent pattern as why they made the change to a healthier lifestyle. Instead of searching for excuses and wanting people to feel sorry for your mediocrity, use one of the following reasons to ignite that fire under your ass:

1)   Revenge (Personal vendetta/break ups or being dumped/getting cut from a team)
2)   Health concerns (high blood pressure, diabetes or unexpected death)
3)   Someone or something inspires you (someone in great shape or as with my redneck roommate, a hunting trip.)
4)   Freedom of time: Retired, kids go off to college, etc.

Revenge
We have all been there: cut from the basketball team, dumped by the love of your life, been called a roller pig by the neighbor kid, or stood up on a date – it sucks! You know what doesn't suck? Revenge.

I have heard a lot of amazing quotes in my life, but the best one comes from my pops. After being called a big pussy by the brothers for being hung-up over what my father referred to as a "borderline of an ex-girlfriend", he interjected in and said, "Stop pouting and turn your emotional pain into physical pain" - brilliant! I am not one to get hung up over a breakup, but when my heart was broken I listened to those words and turned to exercise. It has only been twice, so relax and stop analyzing me you ass-clowns. Sorry, I'm not bitter; I just don't speak highly of ex-girlfriends. Most of them are hookers whom I hope marry short douchbags with tiny peckers, get abducted by aliens, and become science experiments entailing donkeys... you get the point. Like I said, I can be a prick. Moreover, I lived and learned from my mistakes and pressed forward. With the help from my parents, brothers, friends, Rocky Balboa, Eric Church, Colt Ford, and Justin Moore, I moved on. I inspire for perfection with physical prowess, and some of my best workouts came after breakups. The emotions at times were overwhelming. If I didn't exercise, I would have been one angry, depressed, pathetic dip-shit! Look at an extreme example with some boxers and MMA fighters whom grew up in crappy living or social situations. They used physical pain to escape whatever emotional burdens they were carrying. Some of the best fighters and athletes today grew up in the worst of ways. For all of you nerds out there, look at Captain America. He had the heart the size of Texas, but was constantly scrutinized for being a pip-squeak. He used all of the bantering as ammo to become a Super Hero. So what if he used super steroids; whatever, the analogy still works. You need to turn all of your hardships and emotional baggage that you have gone through in junior high, high school, college, relationships, family, life, and work into fuel for your workouts. Why do you think I listen to country music when I exercise? Songs about crazy ex-girlfriends reignite emotions to fuel a fire to be relinquished during the ass-kicking workouts. That fire allows me to press more weight, run faster laps around a track, and do more reps. Use what you consider life's cruelties to fuel your fire and press forward for physical dexterity. Not good enough for someone? Been stood up? Used for sex? Taken advantage of because you are too nice? Whatever kind of pity party you want to throw, go take it out in the gym or whatever type of high intensity exercise tickles your hairy parts. Turn your emotional pain into physical pain. Bottom line, revenge can be sweet, especially when you look better than your ex.

Health Concerns
Unfortunately, a major contributor for beginning an exercise program is a health concern. Show Up Fitness had many clients come in because someone passed away due to coronary heart disease, or has diabetes, osteoporosis, and many other life threatening diseases. My sexy ass girlfriend smoked for three years. As a trainer, she knew she couldn't be hypocritical and tell them to be healthy if she was the one puffing on the cancer sticks. She stopped cold turkey. Success stories like hers are awesome to hear. It is possible to make a change. You just have to accept that you're in control.

One student of mine knew it was time to address his weight issues after he ate his fourth piece of cheesecake and lost his vision for more than thirty minutes - fuck that! Talk about an overwhelming rush of emotions and anxiety. He told himself that he didn't want to choke down pills everyday so he adjusted his eating and exercise regularly. He was able to beat diabetes.

One client had hypertension (high blood pressure) and was taking medication. When the pressure exceeds 140mm Hg and/or 90 mm Hg it's essentially the equivalent of your heart being a ticking time bomb - hers was over 180. We suggested a modification of diet and exercising regularly with us. After three months, she was able to consult with her doctor and go off her meds.
These are just three success stories; I want to hear many more. Whatever your vice or health concern is, use it to challenge yourself to become healthier.

Someone or Something Inspires You

Why do fitness magazines make so much money (besides the horrific advertisements)? The images inspire people to want to change*. The girls and guys are admirable. It's the first step into wanting to achieve what they have. Find someone who inspires you to change. Post them on the background of your phone or computer. Put up pictures on the mirror, car, and refrigerator. I respect the desire to change, but action is required. Implement these workouts and diet plan and you'll get to where you want to be. My job is to find you that little extra piece of motivation. If you need to sign up for an event like a 10k or some sort of race, then do it. There is nothing more inspiring than being surrounded by a gang load of people with the same goals. *Understand that magazines are airbrushed. Watch "Bigger Stronger Faster" and see how they transform the main character via Photoshop. I know it's inspiring to see those amazing bodies, but they do receive help from our good friend Mr. Technology.*

My redneck roommate is a great example of finding something for motivation. He goes on these deliverance-like hunting trips and needs to drop some pounds from his drinking habits. We're from Chico, we can drink with the best of them. In February 2013, I implemented the workout portion of the VTD for him and in three months he lost more than 15 lbs. of fat. He is in way better shape and actually has some muscle. He is even a little cocky; he dubbed the summer of 2013 the summer of SONS - Summer of No Shirts. I find this example perfect to counter the argument that fat loss is 80% diet. He doesn't eat that poorly, but he doesn't eat well. He will have nachos and sandwiches whenever he pleases. He drinks like a fish, but has never counted a calorie or fretted over the saturated fat in the nacho cheese sauce for his elk nachos. Why doesn't he have high cholesterol, blood pressure, or triglycerides levels? You may argue genetics, but I will bet that it's the working out with weights 4-5 times a week. I chuckle when we get home from the gym. The first thing that he does is crack open a beer, put in a dip of Red Man and turn on the Giants baseball game. Hard work pays off. I give him all the credit in the world for pushing his once fat ass, into the best possible shape for his trips - way to go Jacko aka Squirrel. Jacko's my best friend, I can give him shit.

Whereas Jacko focused primarily on exercise, there is another great story of a client and his girlfriend. While he was going through the VTD, she was able to lose over ten pounds of fat by changing only her diet. She was eating no grains, more fruits and vegetables, and replacing soda with water. These are two great stories about fat loss by implementing just one part of the system: nutrition or exercise. Just imagine their results if they would have implemented both.

While we are on the topic of inspiration, I think it's only fair to mention that you will encounter people who try to hold you back. Family members, friends, and even your significant others may hold grudges because of your new health endeavors, so be aware. If you find yourself surrounded by a bunch of naysayers, then try and find some positive influences. Why don't you become the inspiration for a family member, friend, or coworker and have them do the plan as well? I will say that during my four years of teaching, I have had more than nine students go through a divorce during or immediately after the completion of class. Some people may be set in their ways, don't let them hold you back. Do what you have to do to become healthy.

Freedom of Time

Last but not least, people change and become healthy because the freedom of time exposes itself i.e., retirement. The biggest excuse I hear is, "I'm too busy", but what about when retirement comes to fruition? You will have all the time in the world to exercise - no more excuses now. What about when your teenagers head off to college or move out? It's important to realize that with exercise, it's never too late to start. The benefits of exercise will always remain the same: stronger bones, healthier heart, better body composition, and a decrease in mortality. Oh yeah, I forgot about an increase in energy which means more bumping uglies! No matter what age, you can always reap the benefits of exercise.

My parents live in a neighborhood with many retirees. Every morning I see a flock of people beginning their morning walk - that is great! Unfortunately, more is needed. Are you ready to get your panties in a bundle? Walking isn't exercise. It's something that we should be doing regularly. Through evolution, we have evolved into non-walking creatures. As cavemen, we walked everywhere and we should aspire to the same today. Walking to the store, gym, and running errands. Is that the case in the States? I don't think so. An observation my father made when he was visiting my brother Mike in Russia, was "People are skinny, Americans are fat!" After talking with the locals, it is very common for local folk to walk two to three miles to the store; five miles to work. Remember, this is Russia, the walking is done no matter the climate. We should be walking everyday on top of our regular workout routine with weights and high intense cardio. Walking doesn't strengthen your bones or build power muscles. Weight training does. I'm not saying walking is bad, it's just something we should already be doing. If you walk regularly, that's awesome, but you need to start using resistance. Walking is great in the morning, after dinner, for beginners, for injuries, for heart attacks, or after a workout to maximize fat loss. If you don't want to listen to a young buck tell you how to spend retirement, then read the book *Younger Next Year* by Chris Crowley and Dr. Harry Lodge.

S.P.I.N.E.™: Injuries

Granted, I would look amazing in an oversized white lab coat, but I am not a physical therapist, doctor, or chiropractor. This portion of the S.P.I.N.E.™ will be terse and left for proper referral to the designated professional. I consistently hear and see trainers overstepping their boundaries and practicing outside of the scope of a personal trainer. We have the amazing opportunity to help others live better lives, but Pandora's Box is definitely within reach. If a client comes in with a rotator cuff tear (four small muscles that stabilize the shoulder) our job as trainers doesn't change. We implement a proper program to help our client achieve his/her goals in a safe and timely manner. We may give them some exercises to strengthen the shoulder capsule, but in the end, therapists are the ones well versed in rehabilitation. It would be extremely easy and inappropriate to tell the client that we can make his/her injury better. Additional certifications such as a corrective exercise specialist (CES) may be achieved to better equip the trainer with addressing muscular imbalances and elementary injuries.

One of the first tests that I perform on a new client is an overhead squat assessment. Through this movement test, I am able to determine muscles that are potentially overactive (tight) or underactive (weak). I can then implement appropriate stretching and foam rolling techniques to improve flexibility and relieve tightness. Proper corrective exercises will also be utilized to strengthen weaker muscles. Using these techniques, we may be able to reduce pain throughout the body. This is the extent of my job as a personal trainer, not fixing any current or old injuries. By using these corrective strategies, we may completely assuage pain, but that doesn't mean we are physical therapists. That just means we did our job well. Capise?

Injuries can be limiting in many different ways. A sprained ankle may keep you off your feet for a few days or even weeks. Leg exercises or any type of cardio may be jeopardized. A client with low back pain will probably resort to inactivity and bed rest in hopes for recovery. Ironically, exercise alleviates a lot of pain and will accelerate the healing process. People who report having bone and/or joint problems, such as arthritis, claim to have a pain-relieving effect similar to that of a pharmacological intervention when they exercise. In laymen's terms? Stronger muscles and bones translate to a lesser degree of pain. The old prescription of bed rest is no longer efficient, but exercise is.

The likelihood of a client coming into Show Up Fitness without any sort of nagging or reoccurring injury is low. Ankle sprains, Plantar fasciitis, ACL tears, low back pain, elbow tendonitis, you name it, we've worked with it.

One of the best things you can do to prevent injuries is to strengthen your muscles and bones. You'll notice that the first four weeks of the program, consists of higher reps and lighter weights. The reason we suggest this is because it allows your connective tissue (tendons, ligaments, and fascia) to strengthen progressively. Your muscles can handle the workload and stress, but your connective tissues take longer to adapt. It's imperative to all this initial three to four weeks of lighter weights so an overuse injury doesn't occur. Popular programs that you see advertised on TV progress too fast and are too intense for the average overweight person, which make the body more prone to injuries. I know we see all of the success stories via the infomercials, but I wonder how many people were injured through the process. With the VTD, my main goal is to help you achieve your goals in a safe and proper manner.

Some suggestions on preventing injuries and/or treating current ones:

1. Strengthen your weak muscles. It's safe to say your glutes (butt) and core need strengthening. Hip thrusters, lunges, step ups, and squats will address weak glutes, while planks and crunches will target the weak core.
2. Ice and heat. For now, most therapists are still suggesting ice as the primary treatment to keep inflammation down. Heat will open up the blood vessels (vasodilation) allowing rich nutrients to aid in the healing process. Spending time in a spa and moving the injured area may help it recover faster.
3. Be cautious of drugs. Pain relievers only mask the injury. How do you know if you have pain if your brain is being misled? I strongly suggest not taking any drugs before working out because you won't know if pain is truly present.
4. Compress injuries. Kelly Starrett, a physical therapist out of the Bay Area and popular Crossfit advocate, suggests Voodoo floss. As with anything in life, I am a believer in not passing judgment until you have tried it at least once. The one exception to that rule, anything entering my butt. Sorry, not happening. Anywho, flossing is a technique used by constricting blood flow to the injured area. A band is tightly wrapped around the area while movement is applied. Once removed, re-perfusion of blood flows back into the area flushing away cells that make the inflamed area worse. Check out www.mobilitywod.com, Kelly is one smart cat.
5. Rest when needed. Notice week seven of the workout is referred to as a detraining week. Rest is super important for proper recovery and regeneration of new cells. I know it's hard to take time off, but it's necessary. I suggest once every three months taking five to

seven days off. During that time, feel free to walk or go on hikes, but avoid any type of exhaustive resistance training. If this is too challenging, try taking a week off of lower body and then flip-flop and rest your upper body the following week. You'll be shocked when you return to increases in strength and your body will feel amazing! Another trick during the detraining week is perform reps at a percentage of what you are capable of i.e., I can bench press 225lbs x 12 reps for 5 sets, but during my detraining week, I would only perform 225 x 6 reps for 3 sets. A week of training like this will allow the central nervous system to recuperate.

6. When in doubt, refer out. This not only goes for personal trainers, but if you are uncertain about an injury, go get it checked out by a professional! Enough said.

How to fix your S.P.I.N.E.™:

Stress/Sleep- Go to Barnes and Noble or any bookstore once a month. Bring a snack - you can easily spend an afternoon there. I challenge myself to read three books at a time. One on exercise, another on business, and a fun personal book (currently I just started reading "How to find the clit for Dummies- it's a good one!) Challenge yourself to improve not only physically, mentally and spiritually as well. Ask the person at the help desk for the best books on sleep, sex or business; that should get you going.

Psychology- Volunteer somewhere. Hands down the best day of the week for me is Thursday. Show Up Fitness trains a group of special needs students for an hour. If I am ever feeling down or ungrateful, my mood does a 180 because of this awesome group of people. I have never met so many thoughtful, caring and happy individuals in my life. It just takes one simple "how are you today, Chris?" And I am swept off my feet. The world needs more awesome people like them. Thank you guys for being who you are and who we should inspire to become. Good deeds make us feel better and more positive about the world. If you start the good deed, someone else will continue it.

Injuries- Shin Splints aka Medial tibial stress syndrome is a nasty pain that has stricken many of us. Usually dubbed an overuse syndrome from running on hard surfaces and/or tight calves. This injury does not have a quick fix. The best remedy is rest, but highly unrealistic. Try foam rolling your calves and stretching them 2-3x a day for 30 seconds each. Keep a baseball or lacrosse ball at your desk and roll your arches of your feet over it for 5-10 minutes. Lastly, try to offset your tight calf muscles by strengthen your anterior tibialis (front shin muscle.) You can do this by tapping your toes for 15-20 reps while at your desk.

Nutrition- Finger foods. Snap peas, carrots, cut up bell peppers with hummus, homemade beef jerky, pumpkin seeds, and trail mix. These are all great substitutes for you fat finger folk who slam down the chips, cookies, and rice cakes and think you're doing your frame justice. Remember serving sizes! One serving size for almonds is roughly a handful or between 16 and 23 almonds (remember it's All-mond when it's on the tree and when it falls down, it loses its L to become Am-ond, for all you city slickers out there.

Exercise- During your next TV smut fest that you indulge in, perform push-ups and hip thrusters during commercials. You should strive for two sets during the breaks. During a 30-minute TV show you can easily conquer six total sets. This way you will achieve nice arms and a rockin' ass faster than those stupid abductor/adductor machines at the gym.

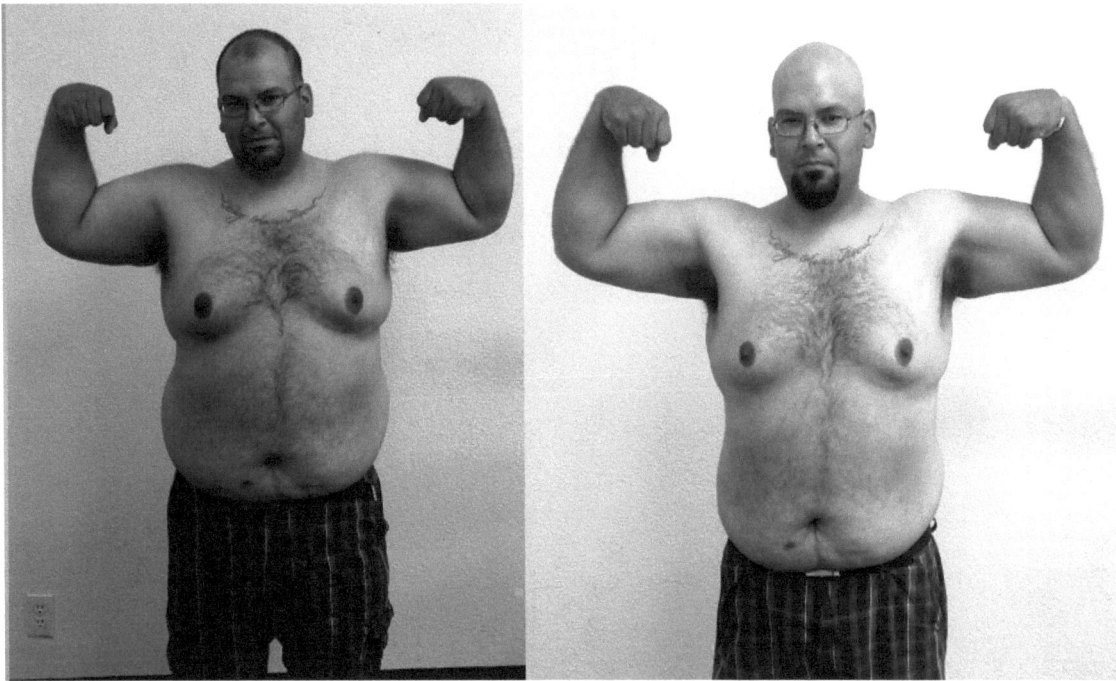

Client 3:

Beginning weight: 290lbs @ 35.1% body fat
Total S.P.I.N.E.™ score of 9

Results after 12 weeks:
248lbs @ 24.7% body fat (lost over 40lbs of fat)
Lost over 20 total inches
Total S.P.I.N.E.™ score after 21

Comments:
<u>Diet</u>: "It was simple to follow and I still ate a lot of foods that I love. The hardest part was giving up the bread. It seems like everything goes well with bread!"
<u>Favorite cheat:</u> "Sushi! I didn't feel bad because everything is so small and still somewhat healthy!"
<u>Biggest success story</u>: "Everyone has their different reason for getting fit, but mine was family and being able to put my socks on without breaking a sweat or hearing something pop. Now I feel like I can take on any challenge!"
*SIDE NOTE. Client 3's girlfriend lost over 10lbs from eating the same things that he was through the diet portion.

Chapter 5

S.P.I.N.E.™: Nutrition

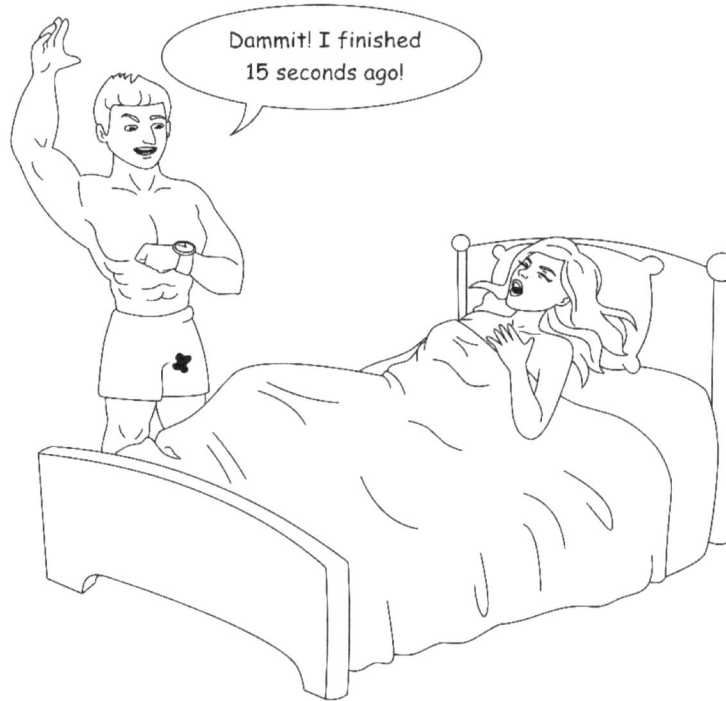

U.S. History: One Fat Nation, Under God...

- 1492: Native Americans discovered Columbus lost at sea.
- 1507: The term "America" is first used in a geography book.
- 1600: A 2-lb. standard-sized loaf of bread cost about 2 pence (three pennies!)
- 1612: Tobacco was first planted in Virginia.
- 1614: Pocahontas and John Rolfe did the horizontal polka and got married.
- 1692: The Salem witch trials occurred in Massachusetts. More than 200 people were accused of practicing the Devil's magic, and roughly 20 were executed.
- 1775: American Revolutionary War.
- 1776: Jefferson wrote the Declaration of Independence.
- 1790: The year of the first census, U.S. population: 3,929,214.
- 1799: George Washington's whiskey distillery produced 11,000 gallons of whiskey.
- 1828: During the election, Andrew Jackson's opponents got feisty and called him a jackass. He adopted the image for the Democratic Party.
- 1836: 39 Americans died defending The Alamo.
- 1865: End of the Civil War. Confederate veteran and American pharmacist, John Pemberton, invented Coca Cola.
- 1894: The USDA's first nutrition guidelines were published by Dr. Wilbur Olin Atwater as

a farmer's bulletin.

- 1916: A new nutrition guide, *Food for Young Children*, was published by Caroline Hunt.
- 1918: WWI. The term "dogfight" originated during this war.
- 1937: John D. Rockefeller died. He was worth $1.4 billion. $190 billion in today's currency.
- 1943: The Basic Seven Foods were established:
    - 1. Green and yellow vegetables
    - 2. Oranges, tomatoes, grapefruit (or raw cabbage or salad greens)
    - 3. Potatoes and other vegetables and fruits
    - 4. Milk and other dairy products
    - 5. Meat, poultry, fish, or eggs
    - 6. Bread, flour, and cereals
    - 7. Butter and fortified margarine (with added Vitamin A)
- 1950: Diet Heart Hypothesis Developed
    - Ancel Keys scared the American society like Steven Spielberg did with sharks in the ocean. His conclusions claimed saturated fats and tropical oils cause heart disease. His hypothesis pushed us toward grains and vegetable oils. (Side note: the ocean still freaks me out. Remind me to send Spielberg a big pile of shit as a big "thank you" present.)
- 1956 – Basic Four Food Groups Introduced
    - 1. Vegetables & Fruits
    - 2. Meats
    - 3. Milk
    - 4. Cereals & Breads
- 1973: End of Vietnam War.
- 1974: First issue published of Hustler (Thanks for all the smut, Harry!)
- 1983: A badass was born.
- 1984: Food Guide Pyramid developed.
- 1990: Robert Matthew Van Winkle aka Vanilla Ice released arguably one of the best rap songs ever: "Ice Ice Baby."
- 1998: President Bill Clinton was impeached for eating a cigar.
- 2006: U.S. population hits 300 million.
- 2011: My Plate was introduced.
- Today: We are one fucking fat society.

How Celebrityville Has Mind-fucked the Shit Out of Us!
I have a joke for you.

Q: When did the cavemen walk into the pantry and grab a bag of chips?

A: Not once, not never, nope!

Fuck me, that is probably a terrible joke, but if you've never seen Drinking Out of Cups on YouTube you should go watch it. Now. Do it!

Do you get the point? To fix our bad behaviors of the past, we need to stop eating processed foods and looking for quick fixes like fad diets. There are plenty of horrific diet plans that promise the inevitable "weight loss" solution, yet the U.S. is on track for 40% obesity by 2030. That means by 2030, 4 in every 10 kids will be obese if we don't do something about it.

Wonder why that is? Fad diets today work for about 3% of the population because we can't change our fat kid habits in 30 days by setting unrealistic goals. Asking someone to lose 20 pounds in a month by drinking water and eating some hot fucking peppers for the next 30 days isn't realistic.

The amount of stupid diets out there is disgusting. Try this: type the word "Diets" into Google, and you'll get over 58 million hits. Celebrityville has jammed a golden dildo into our ignorant assholes, and I'm going to tell you how.

"Popular Celebrity lost X amount of weight on an apple cider vinegar diet." Celebrities lose weight all the time on extremely low calorie diets, as well as hiring personal trainers for ridiculous prices to train them seven times a week. On top of it all, many of their nutritious meals are prepared for them by personal chefs.

At no point did I ever say that they don't put in the hard work or don't have the discipline. It's called resources, and when you have them, shit gets done. But, the average person struggles to even pay Show Up Fitness trainers $60 an hour. Hell, I even have interns who can train for $25 an hour, and that is still beyond the budget for MANY Americans.

We need to understand that Celebrityville is filled with dumbass outfits and flair, scripts for reality shows, and a totally different life compared to that of the average Joe and Jane. Losing 20 pounds a month is extremely unlikely and could be harmful if done the wrong way. If you want to look your best for a vacation or wedding, then you need to put the work in just like celebrities do, but you have to do it without the resource. I promise it can be done following this system. Adherence is the key.

30-Day Rule
I highly recommend the adage that says it takes "30 days to change a habit." There is no science to back this, and some shrinks think it takes more like six months to address change. In the VTD, we are going to stick with 30 days. How long have you been inactive and not eating properly? For the average person, prime-time shape was in high school or early college. If you are 40, that was more than 20 years ago. How can you expect miraculous results at this age? I want you to be bilingual in Spanish by the end of the month - a la mierda. That's fuck yourself in Spanish because it's not realistic. If you set yourself with grandiose goals, then you need to set yourself up for grandiose failure! I prefer realistic goals and baby steps. Week one of my diet suggests eating one extra piece of fruit and one extra vegetable per day for the whole first week. I have trained many people, and I have seen many people fail. The ones who have succeeded did so by setting attainable goals to be reached in realistic manners. I preach to all of my students, clients, and now to you as the reader: stick to this program for a minimum of three months, ideally, six.

To change American fat-ass habits, you need to buckle down for the six-month VTD ride! And, just FYI, it is not mean to call someone fat if they are technically fat. The definition of obesity is "more than average fatness." I try not to use derogatory overweight terms like tub of shit, lard ass, fat tits, Jabba the Hut, fat fuck, Shamu, Fatty McFatterson, Pigzilla, or Fat Bastard (get in my belly) unless the person is mean or if I'm really pissed because Texas or Gonzaga lost another football or basketball game. Being overweight and/or fat is something that can be changed. If you're unhappy about your body image, then YOU need to make the conscious decision to change it. Don't bitch about it and look for scapegoats. I'm tired of the "poor me" sob stories. If you're fat, get the fuck over it. That shitty label doesn't have to stick around. Own up to your actions. We all have our inner demons; it's time to take control of yours and hold yourself accountable. The VTD is your answer.

Here is a crazy statistic for you: two-thirds of people who go on yo-yo diets (popular diet after popular diet) regain the weight lost within a year, and nearly all of them regain it within five years. In layperson's terms, stop doing the same shit and expecting different results! Now, if you want to keep the fat off forever and be healthy while enjoying your foods, implement the VTD. If you want the thrill of losing 15 lbs., gaining it all back and then some, choose the next popular diet book and go fuck yourself because you're an idiot.

This system works. It's a God honest approach to losing fat while teaching yourself how to change your behaviors. People may not like it because it isn't a quick fix. It's a lifestyle modification, and that's what America's fat-asses need. Telling someone to eat a low-carb, high-protein, 1,200-calorie diet is not reasonable because the average person is consuming more than 2,500 calories a day, 50% of which are processed carbs. We are teaching the body to function using unnatural, processed foods. Fast food isn't natural. Chips aren't natural. Guess what grain products aren't? NATURAL. I'm not going to get all hippie dippie on you, but we're fat because of our choices, and I am going to help you make the proper ones. Here are some steps to help you with changing your bad habits:

- Set small goals. Instead of saying, "I'm going to exercise every day," start with, "I'm going to exercise three times this week."
- Don't try to eliminate all the junk food at once and only eat fruits and vegetables. Give up the soda with the Happy Meal or the French fries with the burger. I need to teach you how to make goals that can be achieved, but what is more important, maintained.
- Only try to change one habit at a time. Instead of saying, "I'm going to quit eating junk food, start exercising five days a week, drink 10 glasses of water a day, start humping five days a week and go to sleep before 10 p.m.," start with drinking one more glass of water per day for week one or giving one more blow job to your husband, so Molly the one eyed monster can get licked. Week two, try to get to bed by ten and so forth.
- Write down a 24-hour food log and circle two foods that you know are bad for you that you can eliminate. This exercise gives the autonomy back to the individual and begins a proper behavioral pattern because you are making the decision, instead of being told what to do.
- Enlist social support. They say you represent the sum of your closest five friends. Some people say rid your life of all negativity, including family members and friends. To me, that's tyrannosaurus rex shit because some of my best friends are dickheads and/or big grumpasoruses. That's who they are, and I love them for it. I know who I need to surround myself with at certain times. I suggest finding new, positive social support systems. Maybe join a running club, moms' club, chamber of commerce, or even check out some online dating sites. Whatever floats your boat!

Someone Please Tell Me What a Diet Actually Is!

A diet can be defined as the kind of food an individual or animal eats on a day-to-day basis OR a restriction of the amount a person eats for the means of reducing weight. This is where we have been led astray. We are basing success on the latter and not the former. We need to focus more on fat loss, which is achieved from resistance training and the proper timing of steady-state cardio. Low-calorie diets and running for long periods of time equate to weight loss. When we lift weights we burn carbs, and then after, we burn fat. When we run, we burn fat and muscle. Look at the difference between a sprinter and a marathon runner. Would you rather be skinny and frail OR muscular, defined, and strong?

Let me make perfectly clear the difference between weight loss and fat loss:
- Weight loss consists of losing fat, water, and muscle. Water is easy to lose: just go run for an hour or sit in the steam room for 30 minutes, and you'll lose water weight. Your clothes will fit the same, and you'll still have fat. Muscle loss contributes to the lowering of your metabolism. This will increase your likelihood of osteoporosis, early aging, and a decrease in strength and immunity. Weight loss = being inferior.
- Fat loss consists of losing fat only. When we lift weight and do cardio properly, we lose fat, gain muscle, and look hot! You will have maximal performance, reduced risk of diseases, and delayed aging. Fat loss = superior aka Awesomeman/Awesomewoman.

A Week in the Life of Chris
We should strive for a lifestyle of making proper choices 80% of the time. The majority of our nutrition should come from fruits, vegetables, lean meats, and healthy nuts. Having a cheat meal here or there is okay as long as our default eating habits are healthy. I understand that no body is exactly the same. Governments and scientists will constantly try to find the magical "one size fits all diet," but it won't happen. What I suggest is to try a plan that works for you. Assimilate to all the principals for 30 days and see what happens. Don't start off by making modifications right away. Give it 100% for 30 days. After that, continue what you liked and most importantly what worked. Then move on to a lifestyle that works for you. The only time that I have lived off the same diet for longer than a few years was when I was sucking on my mom's teat eons ago – thanks for the Oedipus complex, Mom!

Bodies will respond interdependently, so you need to keep your head up and keep on trekking down the beaten path for fat loss. If something works, then stick to it. If the Paleo Diet is working then adhere to my workout plan, and together you will achieve your goals. I highly suggest Robb Wolf's book, *The Paleo Solution.* This fellow Chico Alum is one smart fuck and has helped millions of people. If you're subscribing to the Mediterranean diet, and your energy levels are peaking along with a looser belt buckle, don't change anything!

My own diet consists of high amounts of protein, vegetables, nuts and seeds. Some sample meals during my days are: stir fry's, salads with salsa as a dressing, protein bars and shakes, pumpkin seeds, trial mix, organic apples and almond butter, and tomatoes with vinaigrette, oil and mozzarella cheese. After my workout, I consume some simple sugars, lean meats, and tons of fruits like dates, mangos, pineapples, and honey. During the weekend, I drink like a Mick! I fast during the day and before I go out, I work out and eat a large meal immediately after. I would be lying if I left out my late night Taco Bell and Wendy's binges. I love my fast food when I am three sheets to the wind pissed! I am allowed to perform these weekend rituals because my default eating and exercise habits start back up Monday morning. I have set up specific principals that allow ME to do this.

I don't want you to follow my crazy behavior because my body and work ethic may differ from yours. I designed the VTD diet and workout plan because it will instill the proper behavior, so your default programming will override your times of excessive fun. The VTD is a roadmap for your success. There will be no more blind journeys leading you to Fat Island.

Good day	Bad day
Bfast: protein shake with coconut oil, and greens first (24oz water)	**Bfast:** Omelet with meat, cheese and salsa
Snack: 2 servings of mixed nuts with apple and almond butter (no chocolate or fatty McFatterson stuff)	**Snack:** 2 servings of mixed nuts with apple and almond butter
Snack: 2-3 servings of veggies with 1 serving of meat (stir fry)	Red-bell pepper with humas
Protein shake before workout	Protein shake before workout
After workout: 1 large sweet potato/yam with sour cream & salsa. 1 serving of meat & maybe a banana.	**After workout:** Burrito with all the good shit: rice, beans, nacho cheese, extra meat and salsa
Dinner: 2-3 servings of veggies with 1 serving of meat (stir fry)	**Night time activities:** Muy borracho aka I get fucked up
Before bed: 2-3 servings of fruit and protein i.e. whole pineapple and protein shake or an apple with almond butter and grapes	**Before bed:** 7-11 nachos and then some wild monkey sex. **Next morning:** diarrhea and then fasted cardio. **After cardio:** protein shake with coconut oil, and greens first (24oz water)

I consume between 160-175 grams of protein a day and weigh 196. We probably don't need all the extra protein!

I am not encouraging the consumption of alcohol, orgies or anything of that sort. I am just pointing out that there will be times when humans decide to indulge. When you do, hold yourself accountable and get back on track the following day. Remember, are you in control of your actions or do they control you? Wake up and reminiscence about the night while you sweat it out at the gym. If you throw up, that's your body's way of saying "Fuck You - stop treating me like shit." By the end of the workout, your heart rate will have been elevated enough to wash a lot of those toxins out of your body and you'll be feeling better- guarantee it!

As you noticed, there are no specific times when I eat. I just eat when I am hungry, as should you. The whole "six meals a day" or "eat like a dumbass prince in the morning and pauper at night" is complete hogwash. I am not a pauper and you're sure as hell not a prince, so why should we abide by these axioms? The most important thing to figure out during the VTD is what works for you.
Hormones

Scientists are beginning to understand that proper fat loss isn't about calories in versus calories out. I mean, how can 300 calories from an apple and almond butter be the same as 300 calories of Twinkies? It doesn't work that way. It's a matter of what we are putting into our mouth and how it affects our hormones. Indeed, we need to be mindful of what we are putting into our mouths. Moreover, we need to know what specific types of food do to our blood sugar levels through the pancreas. To understand more about hormones, see the hormone appendix.

Starvation

I constantly say that our bodies have ADD; they freak out when something isn't normal. When we go on a low-calorie diet, we are effectively starving our bodies. Tell me if this sounds familiar…

You haven't been laid in God knows how long. You finally put your foot down and say it's time to make a change. You look online for the most recent and most ostentatious diet that you can find: "Really Stupid Name -lose-20-lbs.-in-30-days-and-have-awesome-sex-in-the-meantime Diet." After reading all the rules and fine print, you mentally prepare yourself for the war that's about to happen: 1200 kcals per week for the next month. Week one restricts all of your carbohydrates (including fruit), but you can eat any type of fat or meat that you want. You lose 5 pounds. Your coworkers are giving you props and saying you look great. You definitely have an extra pep in your step and are ready to tackle week two. For week two, you are now allowed to add in some vegetables but still no fruit because it has fructose, which will make you fat. This week you lose four pounds. Your coworkers are giving you high-fives, and you even encourage one of them to try the same diet. Way to go! You decide to go out with some of your friends, you meet a great guy, and before you know it, you two are Hucklebuckin and doing the dirty dirty. It's a magical week! Enter week three. This dreadful, plateauing week allows for one slice of bread and unlimited vegetables, trying to gear you up toward their "maintenance stage," which is a lifetime. Dum Dum Dum Dum… the scale didn't budge. Your coworkers' emotions have downgraded to "hang in there," and, "you still look great, though." But, you're not a quitter, so you hang in there for the last few weeks. During week four, you can eat whole-grain products, unlimited veggies, and one banana. Oh shit, you gained 2 pounds! The diet is now a failure, and you are super frustrated because you didn't hit that magical number they promised. You stop the diet and go to The Cheesecake Factory and eat 5,000 calories worth of spaghetti, wine, and cheesecake. You sure feel good after indulging and just realize there is no hope, or at least until the next popular diet comes out. So you jot this diet down as a failure and go back to your old eating habits. Two weeks later, you put back on all your weight. Back to stress at work, no freaky sex adventures, and mundaneness.

WHAT THE FUCK JUST HAPPENED?

It's quite simple; your inner ADD child doesn't like the crazy caloric restriction. The first two weeks weren't bad; your body replaced the calories that you weren't consuming from your fat storages. During week three, your body recognized this state of starvation from eons ago as the starvation state. For some, this week could happen sooner (week two) or later (week four or five), but the results are the same. It now begins to lower your metabolism by using muscles for fuel. A cocktail of hormones are released, like adiponectin, which signals the storage of fat (primarily around your midsection). From here on out, your fat is being conserved, and any food that you eat will be stored as fat. Eating less than 1200 kcals for females and less than 1500 kcals for men is too low, so your body just makes an executive decision to keep your fat, get rid your muscle, and not let you die. Now you know why you have "stubborn" areas of fat.

Ever wonder why you never see diets below that mysterious number of 1200 kcals? Only Registered Dietitians can prescribe that ungodly low number, not even doctors can do it. After you give up on the diet, you begin eating normally again, and you store food eaten as fat. In the end, your wild goose chase resulted in a net loss of muscle and gain in body fat. It's exactly what you didn't want! Well, guess what? Chicken Butt! Now, guess who? Chicken Poo! Besides that amazing joke, seriously, guess what? I have the right nutritional system to guide you down the right path for fat loss, hormonal rejuvenation, prevention of osteoporosis, higher energy levels, and constant arousal – not just one night stands.

Let it be noted there are plenty of people who don't need to abide by any sort of nutritional system. They can eat whatever they please and work out twice as hard for amazing results. If this is you, go fuck a Billy goat because your genetics and work ethic is inspirational – kudos to you! Be sensitive and understanding that the average Joe/Jane needs both aspects of nutrition and movement to achieve their desired results. Holy Batman nuts, Chris just said to be sensitive; it's a miracle! I know, I know, but people make the mistake of passing along information that only works for their individual being, not for all of society. The VTD will work for millions, not just one individual, so go suck a baboon's ass!

Steps for Nutritional Success

I love asking my students the question of when the average person was in the best shape of their life. The average response is high school and early college before the freshman 15. How long ago was that? Five, 10, 20 years? You have treated your body like the neighborhood tramp, and yet you expect it to be perfect within six weeks. Now that sounds fair, right? Sarcasm: expect a whole lot more of it. I am great at two things: playing air guitar on my brother's legs to Kenny Loggins' "Footloose," and teaching people about exercise and nutrition. Here are my simple steps for nutritional success: more fruits, vegetables, and...

Water

With every new client that Show Up Fitness takes on we make it a point to discuss water consumption. Water is second to air as the most important compound that we must have. Ironically, we are a chronically dehydrated nation (this is usually when people take a sip of water). We can roughly go ten days without water before we die. Food? Roughly four to six weeks with some reported survival cases as 40+ days. Mahatma Gandhi survived 21 days of total starvation, minus some sips of water. This easy-to-drink liquid makes up 60% of the human body, 70% of the skeletal muscle, 70% of the brain, and more than 80% of our blood. The second we reach for that glass of water because our brain tells us that we are thirsty, we have already reached a minimal dehydrated state of 2%. It doesn't sound like much, but for a 200-lb. person, that's four pounds of water lost.

Our nation is continually searching for higher energy levels, and many times the answer can be found by simply drinking more water. We rely on energy drinks and other stimulants. The human organism is being inundated with fake energy and a ton of potential cancer-causing agents. To make sure you are properly hydrated, I recommend monitoring the color of your urine. I'm not talking about golden showers or any of that weird shit, so relax. If your urine is the color of apple juice, get your ass to a nearby water cooler and drink up ASAP – you're already at least 2% dehydrated. A light lemonade color is what we are aiming for, nothing less. A bright neon color is probably the excreting factors of some sort of multivitamin or energy drink – sorry to disappoint, you're not turning into Chuck Norris.

Another important reason I discuss water with my clients is because of our metabolism. If we are dehydrated, our basic cells are lacking the fuel to do their jobs. Mitochondria and all of that high school biology vocabulary crap are not going to be able to do their jobs without water. Mitochondria are where adenosine tri-phosphate (ATP) is made, the basic unit of energy. If we are dehydrated, our cells are not going to allow us to lose weight, function properly, or give us the real energy that we are searching for. Water is water. Don't look for an easy way out by drinking diet soda, iced tea, or some other non-water drink as a replacement. Just drink plain, ice-cold water. Try chugging 16 ounces every morning – literally chugging it like you were still in college. Give it 30 days. If you are a complete baby and can't suck it up, then some other helpful pointers are eating more fruits and vegetables or adding fruits to your water for taste.   If you really need some flavor, try some Crystal Light or Mio droplets, but only as a starting kit. Eventually you should be drinking just water without additives.

Fruits and Veggies
Ten percent of the American diet consists of vegetables, of which 9% is coming from high starches such as potatoes and corn. Politics has never been my forte, so if you want more information on why this is the case, go watch *FoodINC*, *Kingcorn*, or read the book *Food Politics* by Marion Nestle.

So, the next question arises, why eat fruits and vegetables? Easy dickslap, they are high in antioxidants. Let's Hot Tub Time Machine back to high school chemistry real quick.

Atoms are made up of a nucleus, neutrons, protons (positively charged particles), and electrons (negatively charged particles).   Atoms usually complete their outer shells by sharing electrons with other atoms, like Romeo and Juliet or Chris and Mila Kunis. They are highly attracted to one another and are meant to hump like rats in a wool sock. This attraction or sharing of electrons makes the atoms more stable for the molecule. THIS IS BORING, HURRY UP, OR SHOOT ME NOW! Sorry, let me get to the point.

What are Free Radicals?
For beginners, they aren't as cool as they seem because they aren't free and not that radical. Normally, bonds don't split and leave a molecule with an odd, unpaired electron; but, when weak bonds split, free radicals are formed. Generally, free radicals attack the nearest stable molecule, and ever-so-politely steal their electron (kind of like the Honey Badger, sneaky little critter). When the "attacked" molecule loses its electron, it becomes a free radical itself, beginning a chain reaction. Once the process is started, it turns quickly into a domino effect, resulting in the disruption of a living cell.

Why Do We Create Free Radicals?
Don't be fooled because not all free radicals are bad. We do create them to neutralize and fight off viruses and bacteria. Bad things can happen when certain environmental factors, such as pollution, radiation, cigarette smoke, and herbicides spawn free radicals. This is worse when

coupled with the stress of alcohol.

How Do We Protect Ourselves from Free Radicals?
In a normal, healthy body, one can fend off free radicals through antioxidants with proper nutrition and regular exercise. However, if antioxidants are unavailable, or if the free-radical production becomes excessive, damage can occur.

What are Antioxidants?
Antioxidants neutralize free radicals by donating an electron. You can find high amounts of antioxidants in vitamins C and E, as well as in fruits and vegetables.
Wow, are you saying I can combat sickness and aging by eating wholesome, rich in color fruits and vegetables? YEOP!

Here is another brain buster: exercise may even purge these creepy little critters out of our systems more effectively than antioxidants! The VTD suggests that a well-balanced nutritional plan that includes fruits and vegetables, such as kale, spinach, red, yellow, and orange bell peppers, broccoli, mushrooms, onions, grapefruit, pineapple, oranges, berries, and bananas.

Protein
Protein is an essential macronutrient for muscle building, tissue repair, oxygen transportation in the blood (iron), skin and hair health, and thermogenesis. It is essentially the backbone for hormones and enzymes. Most food sources that are high in protein are also rich in B vitamins (niacin, thiamin, riboflavin, and B6), vitamin E, iron, zinc, and magnesium. The biggest advantage of consuming more protein is the increase in satiety (fullness).

A large problem people have with restrictive diets is that they are constantly hungry and psychologically unable to control hunger. They are able to curb their hunger sensations for a few weeks, but after a while they give in. People who eat at least 25 grams of protein for breakfast lose fat more efficiently and permanently than those who don't. I suggest waking up and having a Whey protein shake, bacon and eggs, apple and almond butter, or a hearty meat and vegetable omelet.

Some good proteins are the following: salmon, whole eggs (7g and also the highest quality), elk, yellow fin tuna (30g), milk (8g), and anchovies (17g).

For vegetarians: almonds (9g per ounces), tofu (10g), Brussels sprouts (3g), asparagus (3g), cottage cheese (15g), quinoa (1/4 cup = 6g), pumpkin seeds (1/4 cup = 10g), and last, but not least, semen (1.5g per tbsp).

The dirty dirty on fat

Is fat bad? No. Fat is essential and has tons of physiological functions, to name a few: it composes every cell in the human body, metabolizing cholesterol, promotes blood clotting (so we don't bleed out when we cut ourselves), promotes healthy heart functioning, and is a fat soluble transport for vitamins A,D,E, and K.
Back to Ancel Keys, he misconstrued data and told a big fat lie which scared the bajesus out of us

to stay away from fat. To take a quote from the amazing book TNT* "If A caused B, and B caused C, then A must logically cause C." Right? Let's see if this is true. Sex causes increased blood pressure. Elevated blood pressure increases the risk for coronary heart disease. Therefore, sex causes coronary heart disease. Fuck a Billy goat, because that's not true (thank God!) Well, that's what he did with the science behind his "diet-heart hypothesis." Instead of analyzing all of the possible countries in his study, he chose to review six, but data was available from 22. I don't want to take any credit for this, so I highly suggest reading the book *TNT Diet* (Target Nutrition Tactics) by Dr. Jeff Volek - one of my professors from UCONN, this guy is a stud! Not only in the weight room, (I once saw him out squat some UCONN lineman), but he is super versatile - his Ph.D is in Kinesiology and he is also a Registered Dietician.

The take-home message: don't be afraid to eat fat on the VTD, fat is good. Even saturated fats. Palmitic and stearic acids are good types of saturated fats and do not increase your chances for coronary heart disease. Replacing carbs (other than fruits and veggies) with saturated fats can decrease triglycerides levels and increase HDL levels. We all have heard of these two. Triglycerides are a type of fat found in your blood. Excess calories are then stored in your fat cells as triglycerides. Ideally, you would want your levels to be less than 150 mg/dL. HDLs on the other hand are dubbed the "healthy" type of fat that transfers cholesterols and triglycerides throughout the body. In abundance, these suckers clean out all the bad crap in are arteries, hence the name "vacuum cleaners." Less than 40 mg/dL is considered bad. Here is the kicker. High levels of HDL (> 60 mg/dL) are so good, they can negate higher levels of triglycerides and smaller LDL particles – the "bad cholesterol." Exercise plays a HUGE role at increasing HDL levels, but consuming saturated fat and less crappy carbs can increase them as well. Saturated fats that I consume regularly are found in nuts, avocados, and coconut oil. Coconut oil has 13g per serving and that shit doesn't scare me! This magical tropical oil is also anti-inflammatory due to the fatty acid lauric acid. Additionally, it's really good for your skin - put that shit right on your face, seriously, it's amazing! My face, butt and ball sac feels like a baby's bum!

The Skinny on Soy
"I'll have one skinny nonfat soy latte." Says the 250lb. woman at Starbucks. "Why don't you start off with a small black coffee, 15 push-ups, 30 squats, and a side of jumping jacks for a minute instead, missy?" If only I could have my own VTD coffee shop, otherwise, I would get slapped! We are a society that is hooked on quick fixes. I already debunked your fat misconceptions, now, let me tackle the next popular fad, SOY.

Soy products contain isoflavenes which are estrogen-like compounds that your body processes much like its own estrogen. Not all soy is bad. Let's look at fermented soy, for example, which is usually found in other countries besides the U.S. Foods such as: miso, edamame, Natto, and fermented tofu are fine. Today, roughly 90% of soy beans are genetically modified (GMOs), and, guess who makes them? Watch *FoodINC* and *Kingcorn* and be prepared to have your mind blown. Soy protein bars, soy lattes, soy protein shakes, meal replacement shakes, soy yogurt, bottled fruit drinks, soups and sauces, baked goods, some breakfast cereals and the worse of all, soy formula! They are all poop, pee, diarrhea, put 'em together and get a slushy aka SHIT, SHIT, and more SHIT! Soy contains phytates (aka anti-nutrients) which prevent the absorption of certain micronutrients (vitamins and minerals) such as: calcium, magnesium, iron, zinc and iodine. Consumption of too much soy may also fuck up the function of the thyroid gland via goitrogens. These nasty little critters suppress the thyroid by inhibiting iodine uptake. Holy

Shit, there's more? Soy phytoestrogens are antithyroid agents that may cause hypothyroidism and even cancer! For more information on soy, follow Jade & Keoni Teta at www.metaboliceffectdiet.com and check out their awesome book *The Metabolic Effect Diet*. I utilized their marketing tactic and used the word "diet" in my title as well because people are so attracted to that word.

A student of mine has a sister going through remission. She wanted to get on the healthy train, so, she began taking a very popular meal replacement shake that is soy-based. Just recently, she went back to her doctor for a checkup and the doctor asked her what she's been eating. She told him the name of the replacement shake and he immediately told her to stop taking it. They found slight traces of the cancer coming back. Oh ya, too much soy can even make your hair fall out. It's not your rowdy kids, it's the damn soy!

Do you know when menarche usually begins in young ladies? C'mon people! Menarche is the first menstruation a female has. It's signaling that the body is now ready to start carrying a child, and that's when the menstruation cycle begins. Anywho that sucker usually begins around 12-13 years old in females. Sadly, in the U.S., that number is dramatically decreasing. It's not uncommon for young girls to have it before 10 and even as low as seven. SEVEN! That's fucking insane!

We dip shit guys have to be careful with soy, too, not just the ladies. A lot of our bodybuilding supplements we take have soy in it as well: weight gainers, bars, and shakes. Wonder why you have been having limp dick problems? That little "Iron Sheik" of yours is all of a sudden "Iron Reek" aka your tiny dick doesn't work! Excessive soy leads to erectile dysfunction and a lower humpidity hump hump drive.

Take home message: Be aware of soy that isn't fermented and learn to look for these on food labels (BAD): TSF (textured soy flour), TSP (textured soy protein), TVP (textured vegetable protein) and MSG (monosodium glutamate). For more information, read up at http://www.westonaprice.org/.

Part I in Summary
What works for you is most important. If you aren't feeling results within 30 days, change it up. If you're hungry, eat some fruit, vegetables, trail mix, lean meats, or drink some water. As a chronically dehydrated nation, we are probably just thirsty half the time.

That's the funky thing about diets; they try to be a one size fits all. Newsflash: it doesn't work that way. If it did, everyone would lose the same amount of fat on the same diet. Instead, Person 1 loses 5 lbs. in one month; Person 2 loses 1 lb.; and Person 3 gains 2 lbs. It doesn't just depend on adherence to the diet; we need to consider the rest of the S.P.I.N.E.™. The higher the S.P.I.N.E.™ score that you have, the better the results will be. Human beings are chronically inflamed and are metabolic catastrophes. Our hormones are all fucked up.

The best way to find out what is causing your inflammation is to see your doctor. If you have white coat syndrome, you can try an elimination diet - taking out certain foods for a month and then reintroducing them to see how your system responds. For VTD, the first step in fixing your S.P.I.N.E.™ score will be to take out grains, corn, and white potatoes. For some, you may need to take out dairy, soy, eggs, corn, yeast, and certain nuts to see where your inflammation is originating.

Part 2 – Changing Your Behavior; Weeks 1-8

Here's what you need to do: no more breads, pasta, candy, soda, fruits, vegetables, red meat, white meat, pink meat, fish, or nuts. Pretty simple. Don't eat any of these things, and you'll lose weight. That's what you want, to lose weight, right? Then do that and you will. I'll have you in pure misery and emaciated in no time. Sound like a plan? Now, if any of you nodded your head and said I can do this, please go sit on a cactus and wake up because this isn't possible!

Huge restrictions are catastrophic roadblocks for your mind and body; they set you up for failure. Why subject yourself to pain and misery if tomorrow you could die some crazy death? "Well, I'm not going to die, Chris, because I am special." Tell that to the 25,000 people who were killed by snake bites last year, or the 40 people who were attacked and killed by sharks. My apologies: those are extreme situations. You're much more likely to die from coronary artery disease, which kills more than 600,000 people in the U.S. annually, or the 7.6 million people worldwide who die from cancer each year.

If that made you slightly soil yourself prepare to completely shit your pants. Of those 8.2 million deaths, the majority of them are preventable with exercise and proper nutrition - some doctors claim over 90% of these deaths are preventable with a good diet! That means when people implement the VTD, I'll be saving over eight million lives per year! Schindler saved over 1,200 Jews and had a movie made about it. Hmmm, I wonder if they'll change the image of Lincoln and have a sculpture of me with my awesome beard and sculpted body once VTD goes viral.

The diet portion of this book is simple and easy to follow. It's a two-part system. The first part of the diet plan will teach you proper behaviors like the following: drinking more water, eating ten fruits and vegetables a day, and eliminating processed grains. Once you graduate and you understand what natural energy is, you can enjoy being human. I am not a firm believer of eliminating all the fun foods. If you enjoy grains, chips, sweets, and fast food, then eat them occasionally (or at the right time). You will learn how to do this by part two aka nutrient timing.

Combined with the workouts, I will be fine-tuning your mind to make better choices. Instead of reaching for a soda, you'll understand the value of consuming more water. The word broccoli will no longer sound like finger nails on a chalkboard.

Once we realign our S.P.I.N.E.™, everything will function better: sleep, stress, sex, attitude, pain-free movement, and more. Essentially, I will be turning you into one badass, fat-burning machine! This is when we can diverge and eat what we like at certain times. To enjoy the second part of the diet, we need to address your improper eating behaviors. VTD will teach you how to change your bad behaviors. Think of it like a boot camp for hellish teenagers. In essence, y'all been troubling fucktards and need a basic training ass-whooping!

One problem I have with diet plans today is the extreme number of restrictions they carry. To change this, we need to change our behavior. An example of this can be seen with the Atkins Diet. An average American diet consists of over 50% carbohydrates. Atkins requires followers to consume 20 grams of carbs per day for the first two weeks. This elephantiasis restriction (I enjoy throwing in words that aren't technically correct because it's my book, and I can do whatever the fuck I want) sets up a ton of people for failure. It's like going from making out on the first date to some kinky bondage, S&M shit on date two – it's fucking weird, and not many can handle the change! This doesn't mean that some, including myself, don't mind some weird shit on date number two - it's just not for everyone.

This brings me to the two types of people when it comes to change.

Person 1 (S&M): All or nothing behavior. This takes 1 day. LESS THAN 5% of people.
Person 2 (Non-S&M on date two): Gradually reduce exposure until the chosen behavior is attained. This takes up to 30 days and sometimes longer. 95% of people.

Example of Person 1:
In early 2012, I had a female student begin my six month personal training course. At the beginning, she smoked a pack of cigarettes a day. She was literally a chimney. I challenged her to change her fucking disgusting habit, and the next day she did - cold turkey! To this day, she hasn't touched a cigarette. She had the disposition of Person 1 (or had a huge crush on me, who knows). I put her in the small group of people who can achieve this.

I have assessed, trained, and taught tons of people, and there are not many people like Person 1. In my opinion, I'd say less than 5% of the population fits into this small group. This is my own statistic, so don't judge me, and if you do, up yours! That leaves the majority of people to follow that path of Person 2.
People who are similar to Person 2 need to slowly implement the changed behavior. I am a firm believer of trying something for at least 30 days. This gives the body plenty of time to adapt. Let's use the example of the Atkins plan. If the plan slowly decreased the amount of carbs from their original state, then the body's symptoms would be assuaged, and the likelihood for success would increase.

Example of Person 2:
In 2009, I had a male student who drank 12 (yes, 12!) diet sodas every day. I asked him what type of person he was, and he fell into the category of Person 2. I challenged him to kick the habit by decreasing the amount of diet soda by one can per day. By the end of the course, I had him down to one or two diet sodas per week. He lost over thirty pounds because the goals we set together were realistic.

With this diet plan, you need to look at your past behaviors and make the decision: what type of person are you, Person 1 or Person 2? Either way, you'll be successful by following the VTD system.

What to Expect?
There will be no counting calories, measuring food, or getting rid of a macronutrient (carbs, fats, and protein). The body needs fat just as much as it needs protein and carbohydrates, so why eliminate any of these? VTD is going to teach you how to eat smarter so the body can use the calories more efficiently. The main idea is to detox the body and return it closer to our natural state, free from disease and chronic inflammation. This will provide for a stronger immunity and support for hard workouts. I have had clients lose decent amounts of fat by only

subscribing to the workout plan and others by only to the diet plan. Obviously, the best results come when you tackle them both together and give it your all.

The take home message is, this: don't beat yourself up. If you miss a few workouts or have a birthday or holiday weekend, do what you can do. Pick your battles. If you're going to miss a few workouts, try to be extra good with your food choices. Maybe you have the Fourth of July weekend coming up, and you want to take a few red, white, and blue body shots off the voluptuous bartender's fake boobs. I say go for it; rip that shit up! In the prior days to that event, walk an extra 30 minutes after your workout or do a few extra sets.

My preference is to workout the morning before the party, but that's just me. The outcome is everyone can do this, so shut up with the excuses and Show Up, and the VTD will work.

Here's the Schedule: Weeks 1-3
Increase water, fruit, and vegetable consumption. Changing your behavior is the number one priority. Instead of a bag of chips, eat a bell pepper. Instead of a soda or latte, drink water. During the first three weeks, you'll be slowly reducing your intake of grains, so by the fourth week, you will be completely grain free.

Weeks 4-8
Completely eliminate grains, rice, pasta, tortillas, and oats. Say What? Yes: elimination. Should you feel the need to indulge, save it for after a workout. If your sweet tooth kicks in, go workout, and then have a serving of ice cream. Let's see how well you do at deciphering the following picture…

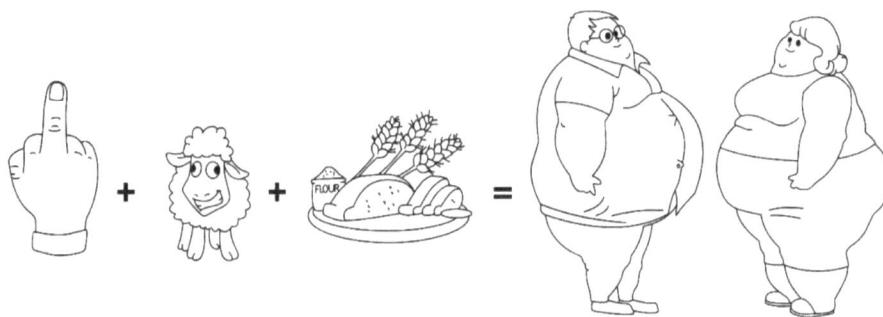

Obviously that's a middle finger. Then we have a female sheep, which is a Ewe (pronounced YOU) and a big pile of grains which equates to a fat fucking nation…

FUCK YOU GRAINS, WE'RE FAT BECAUSE OF YOU!!!!

Choose your battles. If you give into temptation, that's okay because you're human. Pick up with the VTD eating habits the next day. You're default eating behaviors are what will yield the results. Cheats or whatever you want to call them are a part of the game. The difference is that we'll be choosing healthy alternatives the majority of the time.

Your energy levels WILL definitely decrease with the elimination of these foods. These foods are very toxic, and we have programmed our bodies to use these crappy sources of fuel. Replacing the grains with more fruits, vegetables, and water will be the ideal trade off. Think about how long you have been feeding your body these toxic foods. Stay strong and understand this transition is for the best. After we get through this period, we will have optimal and consistent energy levels.

Caffeine has been shown to help with mental alertness. This would be an ideal time to have an extra cup of Joe or tea – maybe even two! Don't confuse caffeine with natural energy. Caffeine is a stimulant, aka fake energy. If we do a bunch of cocaine, that doesn't mean we will have a ton of energy. A ton of fun, maybe, but not energy. It's not energy we are attaining from these drugs – it's mental stimulation. Yes, I compared cocaine and caffeine because they are both drugs. The goal is to re-educate our body on how to function properly via natural food sources. I guarantee that your energy levels will be at an all-time high after four weeks of eating more fruits and vegetables and drinking more water. We're a chronically dehydrated and sleep deprived nation. I'd bet you a whole dollar bill (I am poor) that the energy you're searching for can be directly found in fruit, vegetables, more water, and better sleep.

The Rules
I have two basic rules: 1. Throw your fucking scale away. Better yet, I want you to go into your bathroom, kitchen, or bedroom, and smash that futile piece of shit to shards. 2. Don't give up. Remember, it's all about showing up! Be 100% honest and truthful with yourself, and the results will come. If you put on ten pounds over the past few months, then give yourself a few months to shed them away. If you have gained thirty pounds in the previous five years from sitting at a desk, give yourself half a year. If you've gained more fat than that and haven't been adhering to any sort of diet or exercise plan, give yourself a few years. I know that is the last thing that you want to hear, but it isn't a race, it's a lifetime!

You'll learn tons of secrets and maybe even have fun losing the fat. Clothes will need to be bought. Compliments will come that you haven't heard in years. They'll be an increase in self-confidence, which will be followed by wild monkey sex. Remember to smile. Life is too short to be unhappy with how we look. I am your number one fan and know that if you abide by these rules and don't stray too far from the beaten path of VTD, success is yours to be had!

Week 1: What Type of Person are You?

Person A: All or nothing. Eliminate grains, rice, pasta, and starchy veggies (corn & white potatoes).

Person B: Not-so-extreme? Then follow this 3-week program to gradually eliminate those foods:

Main goals: Water, fruits, vegetables, and eating after your weightlifting sessions.

Water: Aim for half your body weight in water (ounces). So if you weigh 150 lbs., I want you to shoot for 75 ounces. This is the equivalent of roughly six 12-ounce water bottles or nine cups of water in a mug. You may find yourself going to the restroom more, and if this becomes a nuisance, then monitor the color of your urine – aim for light yellow/lemonade color. Gatorade, vitamin water, and other calorically dense beverages do not count. It needs to be PURE water. One helpful pointer is to put a glass of water by your bed, and when you wake up in the morning, immediately chug it.

Fruits: Based on your S.P.I.N.E.™ score, try to consume one extra piece of fruit a day. If you haven't been eating breakfast, this would be the best time to have a banana, apple, or orange. Fruits are huge anti-inflammatory agents, and your bodies will need them during this time of physical stress.

Vegetables: Based on your S.P.I.N.E.™ score, try to consume one extra serving of vegetables a day. A great suggestion is adding spinach to dinner. Carrots as a midday snack or raw red bell peppers are my favorites!

Eating within an hour after your weightlifting session is the best time to consume a combo of carbs and protein. Your muscles have been depleted of glycogen (muscles' fuel), and it's time to fill them up with some carbohydrates ASAP. This is the most opportunistic window to consume some fresh fruit and kill two birds with one stone. Within reason, aka portion control, consider the following suggestions: a banana with almond butter, a homemade smoothie, fresh-squeezed orange juice with vanilla protein powder, or my favorite, two dates with almond butter – AMAZING!

Week 2:

Main goals: Water, fruits, vegetables, and eating after your weightlifting sessions.

The only thing that changes between week one and two is the addition of one extra fruit and vegetable serving per day. This would be a great time for the addition of a salad for lunch with broccoli, spinach, bell peppers, or try an assorted bowl of fruits before bed for dessert.

Still aim for half your body weight in water (ounces).

Week 3:

Main goals: Eliminate grains after lunch AND eat more vegetables and fruit (by now, we should be consuming half our weight in water or even more with increased exercise).

Eliminate grains: No more breads, rice, pasta, oatmeal, cereals, or potatoes after lunch. Grains are tasty, but they are making you fat. The only time it will be acceptable to consume these foods is after a workout or on a cheat day – THAT'S IT!

Some helpful replacements are trail mix, pumpkin seeds, coconut oil with protein powder, and of course, more fruits and vegetables. Your energy levels may decline this week and the next. Our bodies have been taught to run off of crappy starches, so we need to re-educate them. Consuming extra caffeine and water will help with the decline in energy.

Fruits & Veggies: Aim for three extra from your original S.P.I.N.E.™ score.

Week 4:
Main goals: Eliminate grains, rice, pasta and starchy veggies (corn and white potatoes) AND eat more vegetables and fruit.

Elimination of grains and starchy grains: It is known that breads, cereals, and pastas cause inflammation within the stomach lining. Up to 80% of our immunity lies within our gut. We can begin to restore the gastrointestinal (GI) health by eliminating these foods that contain proteins that inflame our bodies. The only acceptable time to consume these grains would be 1-2 hours after a workout with weights or during a cheat day.

Fruits & Veggies: Aim for 4 extra from your original S.P.I.N.E.™ score.

Weeks 5-8:
Practice a lifestyle that contains low amounts of grain, rice, and starches and one that is rich in vegetables, fruits, lean meats, and plenty of water. By now, you should be consuming a total of ten fruits and vegetables per day and you're feeling fucking awesome because of it!

Elimination of grains: Aim for one cheat meal per week. If you get all naughty on me and indulge in more than one cheat meal per week, you're fucked, and you're going to hell! Kidding. I understand there are weeks where there are multiple birthdays, graduations, and holidays. No biggie. Remember, our goal here is to change your behavior and instill a lifestyle of healthy eating and constant movement. Our default lifestyle will be one of healthier choices, so don't beat yourself up over a couple of bad meals.

Part II in Summary
Juxtaposed with the workout plans, these next two months determine your future success with fat loss. The addition of more fruits, vegetables, and water will detox your system and have you functioning at a higher level. I have had clients lose anywhere between 15 lbs. to as low as nothing during this time period. The ones who adhered to the workout and diet the closest had the best results. As I have stressed before, I am not concerned with the number on the scale, but I know you are. Don't judge the program based off of that dumbass number on the scale, but rather on how many inches you lose, body fat percentage, inches lost, how your clothes fit, energy levels, self-confidence, and of course, sex drive!

I had one client lose two inches in her waist, chest, and hips! She lost over 5% body fat and felt great! The scale only read a difference in 4 pounds. Look at the calculations to see for yourself that the scale doesn't mean shit!

At first, your energy levels will decline, and you may even get a cold or two. This detoxification will challenge your digestive tract and detoxing capabilities. Why do smokers cough when they stop smoking? Their cilia in their respiratory tract begin working again by clearing out all the shit in their lungs. Why do cranksters and alcoholics go through withdrawals, fevers, and hell during their time away from the abuse? Their bodies are going through a withdrawal from the absence of the drugs! Giving up grains, sugar, caffeine, processed foods, alcohol, and smoking will all yield similar detoxification results to varied degrees depending on the substance and how long the addiction lasted. The addition of more nutrient-dense foods and water will begin to help the body detox properly. It won't be easy, but remember, it's mind over manner, and keep showing up!

Adherence to the system is the key. If you slightly slide off track, look at yourself in the mirror and say, WAKE THE FUCK UP! That person who looked for excuses was the old me, and this is the new me. I am going to take responsibility for my actions, and if I have a piece of cake or a bag of chips, that's ok because the new me eats well and exercises 70% of the time (that's 5 out of 7 days to all you math stars!) The VTD is not suggesting ridding your life completely of all of these addictive substances, but it wouldn't hurt! The drugs are a no-brainer, but alcohol? Come on, it just tastes so good once it hits the back of your throat! Frank the Tank! Frank the Tank! Seriously though, the results will come quicker and better if you do get rid of these substances! One client gave up tequila cold turkey, and she had some of the best results I've seen on the VTD system!

Part III – Nutrition Timing; Weeks 9-12… (Death)

Congratulations, you have stuck to a new system of healthy eating for two months. Please stand up and raise the roof because this is a huge accomplishment! In the last few months, the foundation for your S.P.I.N.E.™ has been dramatically fixed, and you're feeling the best you have in years, maybe decades.

Your stress levels have been allayed due to better sleep, more sex, and consistent exercise. Your disposition and behaviors have been altered for the better. Your cravings have subsided, and now behavioral decisions are made correctly (instead of poorly i.e. bag of chips). Energy levels have peaked due to optimal water consumption and natural whole foods like fruits, veggies, nuts, and lean meats. For some, this no-grain approach may be your new lifestyle, and it will definitely decrease your chances of morbidity. For others, these past few months may have been hell with the elimination of breads, oatmeal, rice, and pasta. I understand a banal life sucks, so the next part of the nutrition system will allow you to spice things back up aka nutrient timing.

CAUTION CAUTION CAUTION!

If you have been seeing consistent results (fat loss, clothes fitting better, higher energy levels, strength gains, tons of compliments, and you can finally see your penis again), then I highly suggest sticking to the no-grains until you feel like you've reached a plateau. In my opinion, a plateau is inevitable. But if you're still melting off the pounds and seeing great results, why change? I highly, HIGHLY, suggest sticking to part II of the system if you've yet to hit a plateau and/or you are more than 15 lbs. away from your target weight. If you have been reading closely, you know that I think having a target weight is ludicrous (not Ludacris, I wanna get you in the Georgia Dome on the 50 yard line where the dirty birds kick for three), but I know you have one, so let bygones be bygones.

The reason I take two months to even introduce this idea of nutrient timing is because it's a

double-edged sword. As a trainer, when I give my clients or students the green flag to do something, they abuse the power: PIZZA, PASTA, BREAD! Just like The Cookie Monster, you'll eat every carb in sight! Eventually, you'll ruin all your hard work and pack the pounds back on. Many people misconstrue nutrient timing as a means to go back to their old eating habits. If you're hungry at work, you'll reach for a bag of chips. In the morning, you'll reach for a bagel and cream cheese, and sandwiches are suddenly back in the equation for lunch.
No, No, and more No! If you go back to eating carbs willfully, I bet my left butt cheek that you'll turn into a pig. Please don't do this. I honestly feel that through this program, I have given you the skills to understand the next idea, and I hope you use them to maximize your goals. That is the biggest aspect of the P portion of S.P.I.N.E.™. Your psychology and behaviors have been changed for the better.

So, with that being said, continue with caution…

Nutrient Timing
Nutrient timing is exactly what it sounds like: timing your nutrients (mainly carbohydrates and protein) around workouts. If you're an athlete and want to maximize your sports performances, I highly recommend reading the book *Nutrient Timing* by Ivy & Portman. Granted, the information isn't as exciting as this book is, but it's copious and fruitful. They dig deeply into the three stages of nutrient timing to maximize performance and muscular growth. In VTD, I'm going to focus more on the timing of nutrients after workouts, or as they call it, The Anabolic Phase.

During the first few months of resistance training, the main adaptations that take place are neuromuscular – how your brain communicates with your muscles. Of course, some may adapt differently: ASS DOG (remember from chapter 3)! Just yell that sucker out loud one time, super quick. It's like an instant jolt of energy! ASS DOG! Whoop whoop. Wow, I feel better. And I'm getting some awesome looks because people think I have Turrets.

These first few months of exercise have conditioned your body, strengthened your heart, and added muscle (hypertrophy), and you've become metabolically efficient (decreased fat and replaced it with muscle). As you have seen with the workouts, you can do more sets and reps, use heavier weights, and you're not as sore after the workouts as you used to be. We have introduced fasted cardio and High Intensity Interval Training (HIIT). So now, if you truly want to amplify your training program, you should implement proper nutrition. Dr. Hans Selye, an endocrinologist, invented GAS. Not the smelly stuff that happens after a Mexican Pizza, but General Adaptation Syndrome. Basically, all bodies experience the same stress response: alarm, resistance, and exhaustion. During this first phase of GAS, the human body responds to the stressor (in this case, exercise) by producing the fight or flight hormones as well as cortisol. During long duration and extremely intense exercise, cortisol is released in larger amounts and may suppress the immune system. We can limit this exposure to a weakened immunity by eating immediately after our workouts. Whether you're cramming for an exam, scared of flying, being pulled over by a cop, caught masturbating by your parents (guilty, eight times), or in the midst of war, the body will trigger the release of the fight or flight hormones. By consuming carbohydrates you are able to switch the body out of a catabolic response (breaking down) and into an anabolic one (building up). By doing this, you're feeding muscles and maximizing their growth; you're expediting the elimination of chemical wastes and boosting immunity. The window is small (within an hour), so don't waste your time by posting something stupid to Facebook like, "Just killed my legs at the gym!" If you can remember one simple acronym from this book, it's definitely GYAHTEASAFPAAW (get your ass home to eat as soon as fucking possible after a workout).

Window of Opportunity

I'm not talking about the opportunity to have sex after you tell someone the L word. I'm talking about the powerful window (less than an hour after a workout) where our muscles have a predisposition to soak up sugar, replenish glycogen stores, boost immunity, and grow our muscles. Some call it the anabolic window, I say whatever floats your boat, but it's imperative to eat to mitigate the catabolic response and maximize growing muscles. After a weight training session (not cardio or pretty pink weights, but a heavier lifting session) your muscles receive signals from glucose transporters (GLUT receptors for short) to grow, grow, grow, and if sugar is immediately digested - it's really that simple. The signal to store fat is disconnected and cannot be turned on for a few hours. Your fat cells are like the runt of the litter, trying to get some of mom's teat to feed, but the bigger dogs (muscle) are hogging up all the fuel to replenish, repair, and grow! High amounts of the anabolic hormone insulin reduce the stress response of cortisol because insulin is anti-catabolic. Cortisol is a powerful hormone, but after a workout, insulin is much more powerful. As you consume a ratio of 3:1 or 4:1 of carbs to protein, your body will signal itself to immediately start building muscle, while turning off the negative catabolic response. It's important to note that it has to be this ratio of 3:1 or 4:1 and not just high carbs or more commonly, high protein intake. The efficacy of carbohydrates is only superior in the perfect ratio.

Cortisol After a Workout

Cortisol does its job very well during aerobic and anaerobic exercise; it's effective and tidy. When exercise exceeds 60-90 minutes, or if it's too intense, cortisol will attack your muscle and start breaking it down via gluconeogenesis.
(Via= traveling through. Gluco = glucose. Neo= new. Genesis= the origin of something.) In layperson's terms, it steals amino acids from muscle tissue and sends them to your liver to be converted into sugar (wow, see what breaking down a word can do for you!). Who wants their muscles to break down after a workout? Nobody! So here's the quick fix. The greater the influx of sugar, the faster the sugar travels into your blood stream. When we have elevated sugar levels, our brain then triggers the pancreas to release insulin. Check out those awesome drawings in the hormone chapter. You'll see that insulin is like Jekyll and Hyde.

The news dubs insulin as a bad hormone because it is associated with type II Diabetes. This condition is bad, but insulin isn't. Type II diabetic cells just don't recognize insulin anymore because the body was treated like shit. Insulin can be the most powerful anabolic hormone, but if you're a TV slug, it will only grow your fat cells. See, the word anabolic means grow, so insulin grows tissue. Fat is a tissue. High amounts of sugar for a sedentary body will cause it to gain fat and become insulin resistant. When we exercise, our muscle cells are the exact opposite of insulin resistant: they're insulin hungry! Our body sees things in black and white. Sitting on our fat asses all day tells the body to decay, and insulin will store any type of sugar as fat. Carbohydrates are basically broken up into two categories: sugar and fiber. When we are active, like we're supposed to be, insulin grows our muscle tissue bigger, stronger, and faster! Higher insulin concentrations are the equivalent of a protective shield for muscles, guarding them from cortisol's catabolic effects. The example I like to use is a healthy, good looking landscaper who plays the role of cortisol. If you give the landscaper a reasonable checklist of chores to do for eight hours, he will do them. The tasks will be completed in a timely manner, and your house will look amazing! Sounds great, right? Not so fast. Overwork your landscaper, and he will get heat exhaustion. Your house will decay and look like trash. We've all had those horrible neighbors with unkempt, shitty houses that bring the housing market down in your neighborhood. On the flip side, if you don't come home at five to pay the landscaper, he will get pissed off and disruptive! He will start roughing up your house by smashing windows and breaking walls. He'll ruin everything that you worked so hard for. Your insulin! The faster you get home to your hot wife, the better! Moral of this landscaper tangent? Trust your landscaper, and let him do his job. Don't overwork him. Get home exactly at 5 to pay him, and then kick his ass out. BAM. Your house looks great and happy wifey equals happy lifey.

Enough of these Stupid Fucking Examples: Tell Us What to Eat!
According to Ivy & Portman, the ideal ratio would be a 3:1 or 4:1 ratio of simple carbs to protein i.e. 30g (or 40g) of CHO to 10g of PRO. After your next workout, think twice about grabbing that protein shake that has 40g of protein and 0 carbs- it ain't doing shit! Consuming this perfect remedy can help reduce delayed onset muscle soreness (DOMS: add in some vitamin C and glutamine if you get abnormally sore), and fuel the body for the next day's workout without compromising performance. If you like (or miss) white products such as rice, breads, and potatoes this would be your time to consume some of them. I know it is difficult to accept that these simple sugars are good for you, but I promise it's all about the timing.

During our workouts, a hormonal tornado takes place, and we need to stop it. Having half of a peanut butter and jelly sandwich won't kill you. Notice how I said half and not three? Moderation is huge here, people, so don't give your inner little piggy the opportunity to come out and literally pig out, because your results will be lost. Men do have the opportunity to indulge a little more than females because we have more muscle mass – sorry, ladies!

Nutrient Timing suggestions (After workouts):
Chicken breast & sweet potato, oatmeal with eggs/protein powder/trail mix, a banana with eggs, a protein bar or shake (with no carbs), almond butter, banana, organic honey, and white bread, 2-3 dates with almond butter, a Cliff bar (maybe just half), fresh-squeezed orange or pineapple juice, vanilla protein powder with organic honey, sushi with white rice (fried isn't as good), some sort of stir-fry, or a hamburger patty with a white potato.

If you were going to have some sort of sweet or fast food, have it after your workout. Having a bowl of ice cream after a workout is way better than having it right before bed. Getting a burger and French fries after a workout a few times a month won't kill you. When I have a sweet tooth, I'll splurge for 1 ½ servings of powdered Gatorade with my Vanilla Dream protein powder- YUM!

Now remember people, this is not Willy Wonka's special golden ticket to start shoveling whatever the fuck you want into your pie hole. No! You have transformed your body into something that it hasn't seen or felt like in years. Keep in mind that your body is a machine, and it needs fuel. Feed it the proper amount, and you will continue to flourish. I use nutrient timing to maximize my muscle growing and make sure I am fully recovered for my next workout. I eat to prevent cortisol from breaking down my muscle. I want to optimize my immunity, so I ingest food usually within five minutes of a workout, even if I am not hungry. I literally walk out of the gym and start eating a banana and walk next door to my classroom to eat a chicken breast. Sometimes I will order fresh-squeezed OJ from a Mexican restaurant and mix in some honey with my protein powder. Once a month I might have a big-ass burrito or some sushi. But, the next day, I kick tons of ass in the gym.

My three go-to's are usually a banana and some sort of protein, the OJ concoction (which tastes like an Orange Julius), or a sweet potato/yam and fish or chicken. Don't overwhelm yourself with the hour window. I understand that some of you may not be able to eat within this one hour period. Don't fret; it isn't the end of the world. It's not like you won't see amazing results by adhering to the rest of the system. If you have to have grains, eat them within this time frame. I am not totally against grains, I just feel that we overeat them as a society and are not active enough to use all the energy that they provide. If you have to have your oatmeal, breads or rice, this would be your time to do so.

Pac-Man Comparison
During and after resistance training, due to a catabolic state, protein breakdown exceeds the rate of protein synthesis; aka we break down more muscle than we can build up. We will stay in this catabolic state for a while unless food is consumed quickly. This is why it's important to eat carbs with a little protein and GYAHTEASAFPAAW! Waiting a couple hours will not make up for this missed time; it is much less effective. Eating carbs mitigates cortisol release by stimulating insulin. Confused? Let's see if Pac-Man can help.

Remember the game Pac-Man? Yes, you do: that sound when you lose has been drilled into your head forever. Well, if you don't remember, here is a quick Pac-Man tutorial. You begin in the middle of the screen as a yellow mouth (literally a fucking yellow mouth) that needs to eat dots to survive. For fun, you are being chased around by colorful ghost-looking monsters. If they catch you, that stupid ass jingle sounds off basically saying, YOU JUST GOT EATEN YOU DUMB FUCK, HA HA YOU'RE DEAD, IDIOT! If you eat one of the bigger dots (called a Power Pellet), then all of a sudden you can eat all the monsters and get extra bonus points without being killed - it's like a Mario star! Be careful though; after about 8 seconds, your super powers run out, and you return to being the prey. Now, let's compare it to eating after a workout. The bad ghost-looking guys are like carbohydrates, and if you eat them without your super powers, they will kill you, literally. If you time it right, then after you eat a Power Pellet, you can eat the monster guys (simple carbs) and actually benefit from doing so - you'll set high scores!

The takeaway message is simple: with nutrient timing the window is short and sweet, so be careful. Think of it as the cherry on top of the pie. Oh God, I got you thinking about pie. Stop it! Now I am thinking about a Playmate in whip cream and a cherry pie- Dammit! See what you did.

One Day of Fasting (Final month on VTD)
Along with the timing of carbs and protein after your workouts, I also challenge VTDers to do one day of fasting per week during the final month on the VTD (see Fasting Example below). As with the nutrient timing, fasting is optional. If you are happy with your progress to date, then continue as is. The popular term today is "intermittent fasting," which is essentially changing up your eating patterns: i.e. one day or time window without food, followed by periods of eating

higher amounts of food. There are many different forms of fasting: religious reasons, shorter periods as seen in the body building community (8-16 hours), and then longer periods of 36 hours. Some benefits of a fasting period include the following: giving your digestive tract a stress relief, the release of growth hormone, which signals recovery. It also reduces blood glucose levels and maximizes lipolysis (the process of burning fat). One additional benefit, and my favorite, is it teaches self-control. I slowly exposed you to fasting by challenging you to do fasted cardio on an empty stomach. I am not asking you to fast every day, just once a week and preferably on a non-workout day. My challenge to you is the following: on one of your non-workout days, try to fast until dinner (about 5pm). The first time I tried fasting, I made it until 2pm and gave in with a vanilla protein shake, cinnamon, and coconut oil. I withheld the urge to have anything containing carbs until dinner. If you can't hold off until 5, then try eating something with no carbs until dinner. That shake was able to hold me off until dinner, and then I had chicken, a sweet potato, and a one-third cup of rice. Your glycogen stores will be low (the average person holds between 1200-2000 kcals of stored glycogen), so you can have some carbs to fill them up. The goal in part III is to time your meals with carbs and then have one day of caloric restriction. I have had much success with fasting. The reason I didn't introduce the whole day of fasting in the beginning is because you weren't ready for it! I see it all the time. People hop on the "fasting diet fad," and within a few days they crack because they can't handle the low blood sugar, shakes, and lightheadedness. One day a week to maximize fat loss is doable. Here is what a schedule might look like:

Fasting Example eating/working plan during part III – workout around 12pm- not including dinner or any snacks.

Mon	Tues	Wed	Thur	Fri	Sat	Sun
Bfast	Bfast	FC	Bfast	Bfast	Bfast	Bfast
Lunch	Lunch	IF til 3-5	Lunch	Lunch	Lunch	Lunch
WO	WO	NT	WO	WO	WO	WO
NT	NT		NT	DO	NT	NT

WO= Workout
NT = Nutrient Timing
FC= Fasted Cardio (I challenge you to try it one day on a fast, just a walk/get time to clear your head and get some SPI points!)
IF= Intermittent Fasting
DO= Dine Out (Take your significant other out! Have a few drinks, and then go hump like horny high school kids).

VTD Diet in Summary (Parts 1-3):

Phase 1: Basic Training
Phase 1 is the introduction to a new lifestyle. Success begins with education. The first part is to educate you on what to expect. Do you think soldiers are ready for war within a week? Hell no! It takes time to condition their bodies and psyche to be mentally prepared for what's to come. This is what the VTD is doing. The first four weeks are set up to mentally prepare you. I

want realistic, baby steps. By consuming foods the color of the rainbow (green, yellow, deep reds, purples, and blues) we increase the antioxidants in our system to fight off disease. The proper steps will need to be taken toward restoring our natural pH balance and making our body more alkaline rather than acidic. Did you know that cancers and diseases thrive in this acidic type of environment? Other things that induce an acidic environment are the following: drinking, smoking, stressing, not exercising, and not sleeping at least eight hours a night. I have had many students and clients try this workout and diet system – it works. As with basic training, people will fail and give up – it's expected. The ones who adhere and stick to the plan will get the results. The main goal is to mentally prepare yourself to get through the first month.

Phase 2: Ready for War

Weeks 1-4 are nothing too extreme: adding an extra piece of fruit and vegetable per day and drinking more water. By the fourth week we will be closer to fixing your original S.P.I.N.E.™ goal of ten fruits and veggies. The amalgamation of these three nutrients will detox the body and replace it with nutritious food. If you can make it through this first month, then you'll be ready for weeks 4-8. There's no pussyfooting around it; weeks 4-8 will be tough as hell. You could experience lower energy levels, crankiness, low blood sugar levels, and even sickness. Don't worry, I have prepared you for this battle with the VTD basic training.

Grains comprise more than 50% of the Western diet; we who eliminate grains are outnumbered, just like the confederate General Robert E. Lee was. Some may think the elimination of grains is risky, but so was Lee's decision to divide his army and attack the Union army from behind against Major General Hooker. I know this elimination is the single best thing in your battle against cancer, diabetes, coronary heart diseases, and other series morbidities. If you can stick through month two, the results will be a significant victory, just like General Lee's victory.

Phase 3: Special Ops Training. It's time to capture Osama Bin Laden!

Am I still comparing VTD eating habits to war? You're damn right I am! What do you think would happen if we sent off a bunch of unprepared pencil dicks into battle? Mockery and lots of death! I feel too many diet plans do this with the result being diet sabotage! My goal is to properly condition you so you have an understanding of your choices. That's why it's a system. During this phase, we will be introducing nutrient timing and one day of fasting. You'll be allowed to eat grains after your workouts. This will be acceptable because you understand that by doing this you're going to maximize your results (fat loss and muscle gain). By the end, you will know when it is okay to make your choices and not be guilt-tripped. If I were to start off by telling you to eliminate grains, fast, and eat carbs after your workouts you would be confused as hell! Remember psychology and classical conditioning? Okay, you asked for it: Psychology 101 cliff notes.

American shrink B.F. Skinner created this idea that involves applying reinforcement and/or punishment after a behavior. For example, by taking this approach we can strengthen behaviors. Don't confuse classical conditioning with operant conditioning. Operant conditioning was Pavlov and his dogs. He would put peanut butter on his penis and at the sound of a bell they would begin to salivate. Or was that a porno I saw? Anywho, Pavlov was a Russian physiologist who implemented this concept dealing with voluntary and involuntary behaviors based on a neutral signal before a reflex. Interesting shit!

Summary:

You have come a long way. In the beginning, you were eating whatever the hell you wanted and had a higher predisposition to cancer, illness, and chronic diseases. Gradually, you began eating more fruits, vegetables, drinking more water, eliminating grains, rice, pasta, and starchy vegetables. During this time, you became disciplined and understood that you made your choices, not an imaginary gremlin who forced you to smash pie in your face. Nutrient timing can now be introduced because your behavior has changed. You have graduated into a system that can be used for the rest of your life. I suggest flipping back and forth between parts II & III, aka nutrient periodization. By doing this, I see you avoiding a bingeing eruption later on. If you deprive yourself of foods that you truly want, eventually, you'll bust! We have all been there: "I just ate the whole container of cookies and cream ice cream." Then, you feel like shit and will probably have terrible stomach pains. I am a believer in eating whatever floats your boat, in moderation. If you enjoy pizza and Mexican food like I do, then have it once a week. Think of that meal like a track meet. When I was a badass track athlete I would train my ass off in preparation for that meet (I really wasn't, but in my mind, I am a whole bunch of cool shit). During the track meet, I enjoyed myself and had the time of my life. If you take this approach (Part III) with food, you will never have that feeling of guilt again. You earned that food. If you do slip up, who gives a flying fuck? Just get back on track and kick ass the next day. Life is way too short to sweat the small things!

Recipes:

These recipes are made for one fat ass person aka me! Remember, I eat a lot, so you could probably stretch out the recipe for a family of four or yourself for a week. If you're vegetarian, just take the meat out. For more recipes, check out my website, www.Show Upfitness.com.

Chris' Fucking Awesome Sheppard's Pie
   - 2 lbs pound of meat (turkey, 100% grass fed beef, chicken, bacon, sausage whatever you'd like). I typically choose 1lb of grass fed beef along with 1lb of sausage or kielbasa.
   - Fresh Veggies my choices have been 1 box of mushrooms, onion and bell peppers.
   - 3 sweet potatoes
   - Bag of Spinach
   - ½ cup of jack cheese
   - Spices (Sriracha, tapatio, salt, garlic, and whatever else)

1. Cook meat in a frying pan until finished (season appropriately.)
2. Add 16 oz tomato puree and vegetables.
3. Add spices for taste (my favorite is 3 tbsp. of Sriracha hot sauce & fresh crushed garlic).
4. In a separate pan, steam 1 bag of spinach and microwave or cook the 3 sweet potatoes. I usually poke em with a fork to release the steam as they cook. When finished, mash them all together in a bowl. Add pepper and jack cheese to make it super orgasmic!!!
5. Put it all together for the finished product (30-40 minutes)…
6. In a pie pan, cover the bottom with 2-3 inches of the sauce & meat (leftover sauce & meat is for breakfast the next day). On top of the sauce, add the spinach and then top it off with the sweet potatoes.

Chris' Big OL' Titties Stir Fry (3 options)
- 2 lbs pound of meat (I prefer a pre-cooked chicken, turkey or 100% grass fed).
- Fresh Veggies: head of cauliflower, 20+ stocks of asparagus, box of mushrooms, 1 onion and 1 red, yellow and green bell peppers.
- Option 1 HOT: Sriracha, salt, garlic, and chicken broth- homemade is the best!
- Option 2 SWEET: 1 pineapple cut into chunks and pineapple squeezed into pan as a sauce.
- Option 3 Almond Butter: 1-2 servings of almond butter, a little sour cream and milk– tastes like a peanut butter sauce, YUM!!!!!

1. Put sauce in bottom of pan with 1-2 tablespoons of coconut oil.
2. Add veggies until finished, I like to cover wok (10-15 minutes.)
3. Add pre-cooked chicken at the end.
4. OR cook meat in a side pan and add in when finished.
5. Take wok off of burner and let meat soak in sauce for additional 5-10 minutes

Chris' Bonerific Meatatarian Pie
- 2 lbs pound of meat (100% grass fed ground beef or lean turkey).
- 1 package of bacon
- 1 sliced onion
- Spices (Sriracha, tapatio, salt, garlic, and whatever else)

1. Mix 2lbs of meat with sliced onions in a small pie pan (add spices). I am not a fucking chef, it's a smaller 2-3 inch pan – my mom would usually cook her pies in them.
2. Line the top of the pan with strips of bacon
3. Cook the boner pie for 30 minutes at 350 (40+ minutes if you like the bacon more crisp.)
4. An awesome addition is to eat this with the stir fry (just veggies).

Chris' Big Hairy Meatballs (without the hair)
- 2 lbs pound of 100% grass fed beef whatever ground meat you like.
- Bread crumbs
- 2 eggs
- Pepper Jack Squares
- Spices (BBQ sauce, Sriracha, tapatio, salt, garlic, and whatever else)

1. Mix meat, bread crumbs, eggs and sauces into a bowl. My choice is BBQ sauce. If you are afraid of the sugar, eat the meatballs after a workout!
2. Mold the meat into desired size for meat balls. I enjoy making a bunch of smaller ones (2-3inches) and then one big mother fucker.
3. Add pepper jack squares into the middle of each meatball
4. Place into oven at 325 for 30-40 minutes (or until golden brown color).
5. Be aware, these are fucking ORGASMIC!!!!!

Foxy Curry Meatballs:
For a little variety from my Hairy Meatballs, try these ones out for a little ethnic curveball.

- 2 lbs pound of turkey meat (or my favorite... ELK)
- 2 eggs
- Spices: curry powder, oregano, dill and garlic. I didn't measure these fuckers out, just do a little splash here and a pinch or two there. Rules are sometimes boring to follow.
- EXTRA, try this the second time you make these suckers:
- ¼ inch mozzarella cubes to place in the middle of each turkey ball – great addition, but try the original one out first.

1. Mix meat, eggs and spices into a bowl.
2. Mold the meat into desired size for turkey balls.
3. Place into oven at 325 for 30-40 minutes (or until golden brown color).
4. After they have cooled down, take one and throw up in air as high as you can to see if you can catch in your mouth, it's fun.

Chris' Elk Burgers and Chicken thighs (Bulk Cooking)
- 1 pound of Elk meat. One of the healthiest lean meats out there and it's even better when its free because your red neck roommate shot it!
- 1 eggs
- Pepper Jack
- Spices (BBQ sauce, sriracha, tapatio, salt, garlic, and whatever else)
- 12 Chicken Thighs

1. Mix meat, eggs and sauces into a bowl. My choice is BBQ sauce. Boobs, BBQ and Ranch are my three guilty pleasures. Hmmmm, BBQ chicken wings dipped in ranch served by a topless girl = HEAVEN!
2. Mold 3-4 burgers to desired size.
3. Place burgers in middle and chicken thighs around BBQ. They say you aren't supposed to cross-contaminate chicken with other meats, but I don't give a fuck. I just cook the shit out of them to kill all the little germies!
4. Cook until done.
5. Add pepper jack on top.

Chris' Pineapple dessert to add along with the Burgers and Chicken thighs (Bulk Cooking)
- 1 large pineapple. To make life easier, purchase one of the best inventions ever, a Pineapple cutter- AWESOME!
- Cinnamon
- Brown Sugar
- Water

1. Cut pineapple into 6-10 circular rings.
2. Put into one large freezer bag with water, cinnamon, brown sugar and water and place into refrigerator for 30-60 minutes.

3. After your done cooking up the meat from the previous bad-ass recipe, put marinated pineapple onto grill and cook for 2-3 minutes per side.

Jayson's kick ass Honey Mustard Almond Pork Chops
This recipe originally called for bread crumbs, but we are grain free, so we improvised by using crushed almonds and additional spices.
- Olive Oil or Spray For Baking Sheet
- Chop Up Almonds (Food Processor or Blender)
- Garlic Herb Ms. Dash
- Homey Mustard
- 2 tbsp. Sea Salt & 2 tbsp. Pepper

1. Preheat oven to 450
2. Chop Up Almonds In Food Processor or Blender and add all into a mixing bowl with Garlic Herb Ms dash, Add Pepper and Sea Salt
3. In a smaller bowl, add honey mustard and coat the pork chops (you can trim off the fat if you'd like.)
4. Cover pork chops in honey mustard and then coat with almond mix.
5. Place pork chops on a baking sheet and cook for cook for 8 minutes on each side or until golden brown one each side

Ratatouille – like the fucking movie! (Vegetarian)
- 2 tablespoon oil, olive
- 2 clove(s) garlic, minced
- 1 onion sliced
- 1 eggplant peeled and diced
- 3/4 cup(s) pepper(s), green, bell, diced
- 2 zucchini sliced
- 2 tomatoes chopped
- 2 tablespoon basil, fresh
- 1 tablespoon capers, drained (optional)
- 1/4 teaspoon pepper, black ground

1. Heat the oil in a large nonstick skillet. Add the onion and garlic; stir-fry over medium-high heat about 2 minutes.
2. Add the eggplant and stir-fry about 2 minutes. Add the zucchini, green pepper, and tomatoes; stir-fry 3 minutes more.
3. Add the basil, salt, and pepper. Cover and simmer 30 minutes over low heat.
4. Uncover, stir gently, and simmer 10 minutes more. Add the drained capers. Serve hot or chilled. When you're done, make sure to yell "I just make fucking Ratatouille!"

Random concoction
- 1 large sweet potato or yam.
- 1 pound of ground meat
- Sour cream

- Spices (BBQ sauce, sriracha, tapatio, salt, garlic, and whatever else)
- Cheese

1. Cook potato in microwave for 5-8 minutes
2. Cook up ground meat with spices
3. Mash up potato to make as bottom layer on a plate
4. Add meat on top
5. Add spices, salsa, BBQ, sour cream & cheese.
6. Put on Gonzaga or Texas game

Vegetable Minestrone soup with white beans

This sucker has over 10g of protein and 10g of fiber per serving… And it's vegan! Add in chicken, sausage or any additional meat to man it up a tad.

- 2 cups precooked white beans
- 1 medium yellow onion, peeled and diced into medium pieces
- Water
- 1 medium carrot, peeled and cut into 1/2-inch pieces
- 4 medium stalks celery, cleaned and cut into 1/2-inch pieces
- 6 to 12 cloves garlic, peeled and trimmed of root ends
- 1 cup cubed squash & 4 cups spinach
- 2 medium sweet potatoes or yams (1-inch cubes)
- 8 cups (64 oz.) vegetable stock or broth
- ¼ cup olive oil & ¼ cup chop parsley
- Spices to taste
- Additional CHEESE at the end

1 Heat stock. In a separate large soup pot, heat olive oil. Add carrots, onions, celery, garlic, and potatoes. Sauté for 10 minutes, stirring frequently.
2 Add greens and sauté for 5 minutes, then add white beans, parsley, and squash and season lightly.
3 Add hot stock, bring to a boil, then reduce heat and simmer for 30 to 45 minutes until vegetables are fork-tender but still retain their shape

Chris' special Jicama Slaw

If you haven't tried some Jicama, you're missing out! This root vegetable packs a punch with 6g of fiber and is super refreshing.
- 3 Tbsp. fresh lime juice
- 2 Tbsp. coconut oil
- ¾ tsp. salt
- ¼ tsp. black pepper
- 2 lbs. jicama, peeled and cut into julienne strips (8 cups)
- 1 medium red onion, finely chopped
- 1/3 cup finely chopped fresh cilantro

- Pinch of sugar to taste (A pinch, don't get too happy!)

1 Whisk together the lime juice, oil, sugar, salt, and pepper in a large bowl until well combined.
2 Add jicama, onion, and cilantro and toss well. Quick, easy, and nutritious!

"The Chris" Steak Wraps
Why "The Chris"? Because making this will give you Abs and buns of steel like mine! Dammit, tool comment number 3.
- 1-2 pounds of flank steak
- 2 tomatoes
- 1 onion diced
- 1 can of black beans
- 1 giant big-ass iceberg lettuce head
- Favorite type of salsa

1 BBQ up the flank steak. This type of meat is thin so you only need to cook it for 3-5 minutes per side.
2 Chop up all the veggies while the meat is cooking.
3 Separate the leaves or whatever the fuck they are called from the head of lettuce to use instead of tortillas.
4 Thinly slice up meat and dress to your liking. Add salsa and WAALLAAAAA, "The Chris."

I hate it when books only put the healthy choices down, so check this one out... DURING NUTRIENT TIMING ONLY:

Grandpa H's Killer Mexican Casserole
"Killer" as in awesome and not explosive diarrhea.
- 1-2 pounds of 100% grass-fed ground beef
- 1 can of creamed
- 1 can of cream of mushroom soup
- Half and half
- 1 can of diced green chilies
- 6-8 flour tortillas
- Pepper jack cheese
- Sour cream & Salsa
- 1 big ass casserole dish

1 Cook up the ground beef.
2 Cook up can of cream mushroom soup. Use empty can to pour 1 cup of half and half and get all the rest of the goodies out.
3   Add in can of diced green chilies into soup.
4 Simmer tortillas on stove for 10-15 seconds per side to turn tortillas hard. If you skip this step the casserole turns into one pile of goopy shit! I like to put straight onto the surface where the burner is and give it a light brown/black hint.
5 Layer the bottom on the casserole dish with stiff tortillas (stiff as in slightly cooked, not as in a rock hard erection.)

6   Cover the tortillas with the ground beef
7   Cover the ground beef with cheese
8   Pour half of the soup base over = layer 1
9   Cover with remaining tortillas
10   Repeat steps 6-8
11 Enjoy this super yummy dish with salsa and sour cream and try to eat it within one hour of working out! Otherwise, just make sure to have a kickass workout the next day.

How to fix your S.P.I.N.E.™:

Sex- Watch each other masturbate. There is nothing hotter than seeing your significant other please themselves while you watch and learn some new tricks of the trade. Give yourself a timer - no touching for 10 minutes. Testing your self-control will bring forth anticipation that you cannot even begin to imagine!

Psychology- Seems today the world is filled with narcissism. When was the last time you started your day with the goal of helping others rather than yourself? With each act of charity, you'll become closer to the person you want to be. Little things help people. A simple smile. Holding a door. A genuine compliment. Put a quarter in the parking meter next to you. Make someone else's day and watch how much better yours become. Pay it forward.

Injuries- Rest. It's not an option, it's a requirement. If you're a beginner, you probably need more of it. Workout 4 days, rest for 3. After a few weeks your body becomes conditioned and in better shape, try 5-6 days with one day of rest. Your body will be sore and pushing too hard for too long can compromise your immunity. Here is a good rule of thumb. If you're questioning whether or not to exercise when you're not feeling well use the above-your-neck rule. If the signs and symptoms are only above your neck (sore throat, runny nose, or headache) it's probably ok to workout. When the symptoms are below the neck, systemic, body aches, flu-like symptoms, and/or green discharge, it's best to take a few days off. If you push during these times, you can make it a lot worse!

Nutrition- Buy a dozen eggs. Throw in your favorite veggies (asparagus, peppers, onions, and spinach) and meat (ham, turkey, and sausage). Cook it all up in that new fancy wok that you just bought. Put it in a plastic container and look what you just did, made breakfast for the next 3-4 days. Microwaved, leftover eggs are actually pretty damn good!

Exercise- Neighborhood workout. Create flyers, hand them out to the neighbors you like (I know we all have some fucking weirdo neighbors so just skip them), and start a bi-weekly bootcamp. You don't need much. Jump ropes, medicine balls, a few dumbbells, and some kick ass jams. "2 legit, 2 legit to quit!" Download a fitness app (I like Tabata Pro) and set each station for 30 seconds with 15-second rest periods.

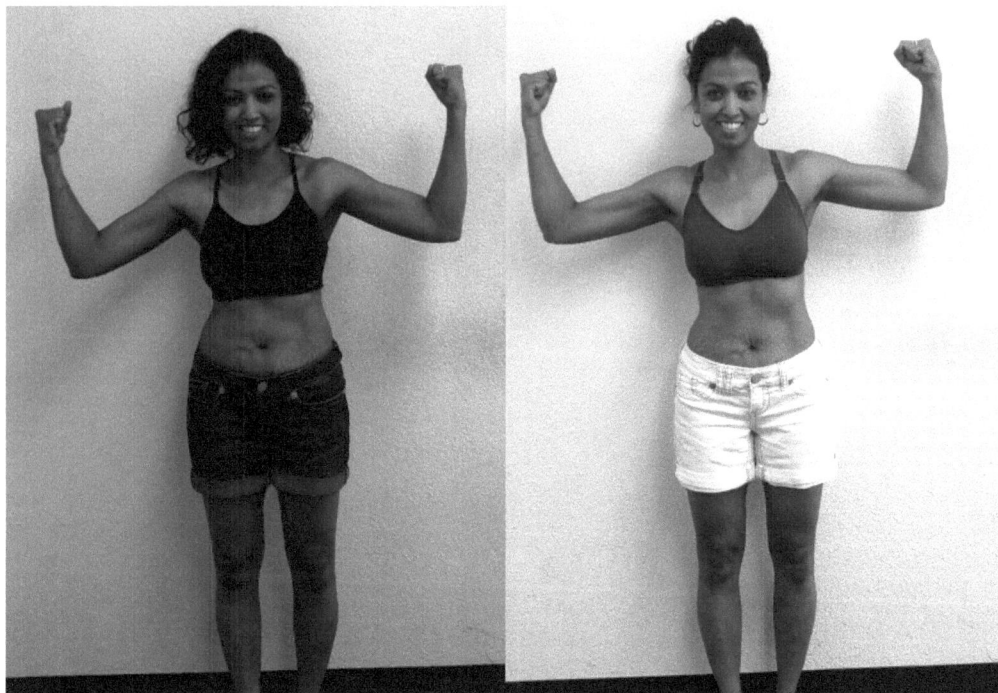

Client 4:

Beginning weight: 127.5lbs @ 24.7% body fat
Total S.P.I.N.E.™ score of 14

Results after 12 weeks:
121lbs @ 20.4% body fat (lost over 7 lbs of fat)
Lost over 5 total inches
Total S.P.I.N.E.™ score after 23

Comments:
Workouts: "The variety of the challenging exercises, there was no chance to get bored."
Diet: "There was no calorie counting, I had tried several diets in the past and nothing had worked out. It was always difficult to note every single calorie I ate. During the nutrient timing portion to eat grains after the workouts, because of that I never had a craving to eat grains during rest of the day."
Biggest success story: "In December of 2008 when I had to get back surgery. Before I got my surgery, I was physically very active and fit. After my surgery however, I was too afraid to proceed with the amount of physical activity I used to take part in; I was always worried that I would injure my back again. All the running, biking and various routines- they were all gone. As a result, I had gained lot of weight. All the work I had put into staying fit was gone. I became lazier, did not feel right, tired all the time, was always frustrated because my back used to hurt with very little activities, I wouldn't look good in my own clothes anymore. Fortunately, I soon joined The VTD challenge. At first, I struggled; it was a challenge to get out of the place I was in. I even started to wonder if it was all worth it. Little did I know that this would be one of the best decisions I had ever made. I began getting used to routines and slowly started to feel good about myself again. I started to love exercise and didn't go one day without it. I began to see some dramatic changes in myself. I cannot believe that I can lift so much weight, take part in so many exercises, and excel so much physically. Looking back, I never would have thought I would be here, and I never would have even guessed I would achieve such an amazing fitness goal."

Chapter 6

S.P.I.N.E.™: Exercise

Holy Shit Factoid of the Day:
When in heat, some Lions may stick it to each other between 20 and 40 times a day for several days (some even reported as many as 50) - HOLY SHIT (WHAT HORNY FUCKING BASTARDS!!!)

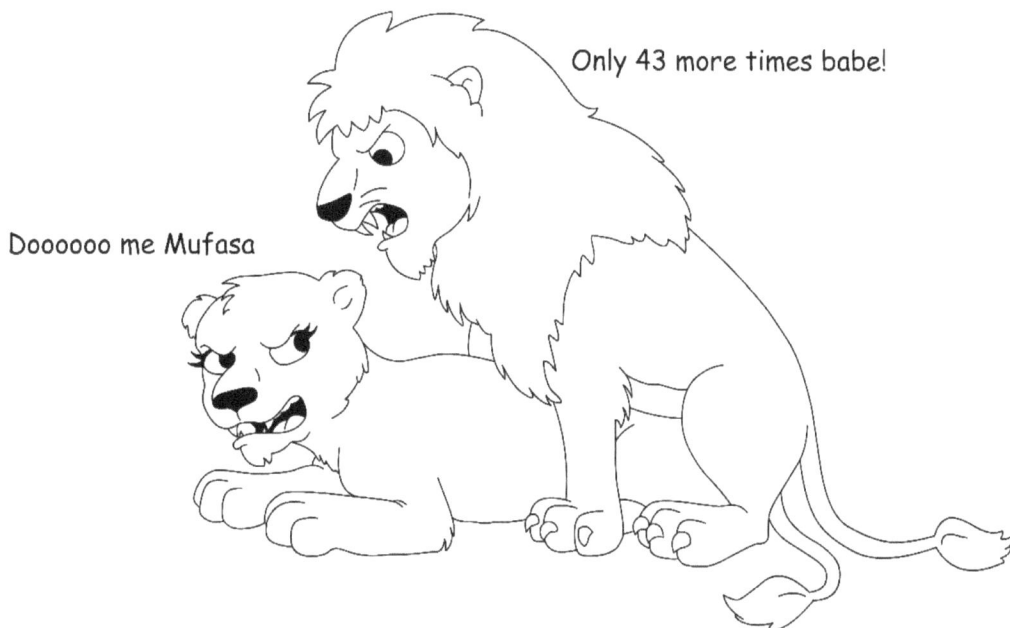

Why do you exercise?

I know why I do, but why do you? They say that the best type of exercise is whatever kind you enjoy. I agree...sort of. We need to find a happy-medium. In today's world, people just don't want to work hard. Lifting weights for an hour isn't the world's easiest task. Instead of working, people bitch and look for quick fixes and gimmicks like the *Shakeweight*, a highly restrictive diet, or *Prancercise*! *Prancercise*? Ohh, Chris, I'm not familiar with this term. Do tell!

Prancercise is when people prance around like fucking horses. I'm dead serious! Who thinks of this shit? Having fun while exercising is important, but it needs to be within reason. I don't care if weights are your nemesis: learn to enjoy them. A good number of people work 40+ hours per week, and they don't enjoy their jobs, but they still show up. If Americans took this approach with exercise, we all wouldn't be so fat. Show Up for 30 days, and I bet you'll start enjoying the results. If you have an injury or medical condition restricting you from using weights, that's the only exception. No ifs, ands, or buts! Women in particular need to lift heavier weights because they're more prone to osteoporosis.

Benefits of Exercise

Here is a SMALL list of benefits of exercise. I am not even going to touch on athletic performance benefits or prevention of sports related injuries; that's for another book.

- **Reduces the risk of chronic disease and conditions like the following**: Type 2 Diabetes, high blood pressure, dementia, stroke, and obesity.
- **Prevention of the leading cause of death in the US, coronary heart disease (CHD)**: Roughly 600,000 people died in 2012 from heart disease. Guess what peeps? CHD can be prevented. Continuous exercise breaks down plaque, and your heart will become more efficient at pumping. When the heart becomes stronger, it pumps out more blood per beat. That means it doesn't have to beat as fast to expend the same amount of effort. Lance Armstrong has a resting heart rate under 45 beats per minute. The average American's is between 70-80bpm. When we exercise, our hearts don't have to work as hard.
- **Better sleep**: When you adhere to this system and begin exercising 4-5 days per week, your sleep habits will improve. Remember what happens when you improve the quality of sleep? Growth hormone is released, which helps regenerate and restore your body's cells. You'll look younger, feel better, and be 100% restored to tackle the day.
- **Healthier skin**: Your skin is your body's largest organ, and exercise helps maintain its youthful appearance. I'd be willing to bet my left butt cheek that you're spending more money monthly on beauty products than exercise. How about you invest that money into working out and see what happens next: longevity and the Fountain of Youth! To top it off, hit the steam room after your workout for a complete cleanse. Make sure to wash up afterwards because bacteria can build up, leaving you with acne – yucky.
- **Decreases arthritis and rheumatoid arthritis pain**: The efficacy of strength training may be just as potent as medication. Water aerobics is all fine and dandy, but where are the weights? There has to be a little discomfort to achieve the desired results. Do you think Michael Jordan's path to greatness was paved? Know your limits, but challenge yourself to carefully push beyond them.
- **Stress release, immunity, and productivity boost:** A healthy amount of exercise combats the production of free radicals. Remember, these suckers attack our DNA structure. Along with reducing stress, exercise will improve productivity. In the book, *Be Excellent at Anything*, author Tony Schwartz highlights mega studies that have been performed on this phenomenon. People exercising regularly, not only work less, but are also more productive. This not only makes you a better worker, it also keeps the morale in the workplace better. Companies with less sick time end up with lower healthcare costs, aka more money for everyone.
- **Bone Health:** Bones are comprised of two major components: minerals (calcium and phosphorous) and bone cells (osteoblasts and osteoclasts). Large amounts of calcium are laid down during our teenage years in preparation for adult growth. In order for our bones to stay strong and healthy, they constantly regenerate. The bone cells work together to break down and then regenerate new bone cells. Osteoclasts eat away at our bones, while the osteoblasts recreate the bones (Here's a helpful pointer: "Blasts" building up, "Clasts" claw down). Depending on your sex and genetics, peak bone mass is reached somewhere between the ages of 18 and 30. After that, our bones do not regenerate in the same way. During menopause, women begin to lose a significant amount of bone mass more than males due to the large decline in estrogen and progesterone. It seems that estrogen plays an important role in bone health by keeping osteoclasts in line, allowing the osteoblasts to build bone cells. If you are a menopausal woman, you can lose up to 7% of your bone mass every year. This can cause great health risks, as your bones are susceptible to breaks and fractures. The cure? Heavy weightlifting. Not the shit you see on Dr. Oz like walking, running, stair climbing, jumping rope, or playing tennis. It needs to be heavy loading on your S.P.I.N.E.™ (squats, weighted lunges, etc). Again, the key is heavy. One of my biggest man

crushes was, and still is, my professor at the University of Connecticut, Dr. Kraemer. He suggests women should be lifting loads corresponding to 80 to 90 percent of maximal for bone benefits (that's heavy weights for 4-8 reps). Granted, you need to start somewhere, so 15-20 reps in the beginning is normal. After a month, the weight needs to be increased to an amount such that you can barely lift 4-8 times with proper form. Those pretty pink weights and black weighted bars make vaginas big, ugly and loose so stop using them – that should scare you away from ever using light weights again!

- **Increases energy levels, serotonin in the brain, and the production of brain-derived neurotropic factor (BDNF):** Exercise can be useful in treating depression. The release of the endorphins, norepinephrine, dopamine, and serotonin have all been shown to help to reduce depression. How can large pharmaceutical companies make money off of this recommendation? They can't; that's why we don't hear about it. BDNF is a protein that plays a role in neuroplasticity, specifically the growth and survival of new nerve cells. A nice stroll in the park will not suffice. The duration and intensity needs to be high. Check out Naperville Central High School in Illinois. There is an option for some students to take a morning PE class. In the recent years since that program began, the students who signed up for PE directly before English or Math showed dramatic improvements in their standardized testing. Take-home message for all you parents out there: Have your kids go play outside for 30 minutes before they begin their homework. Watching TV and playing video games just makes your kids fat and stupid.

- **Increased metabolism:** Muscle weighs more than fat, right? No. One pound of fat is the same as one pound of muscle; it's the volume that differs. One pound of fat is about the size of a softball, while one pound of muscle is the size of a baseball. The more muscle we have, the higher our resting metabolic rate will be, aka burning calories at rest. The more muscle that you put on from resistance training makes you better at burning fat; we literally transform into fat burning machines! In layperson's terms, cheating with a cookie or bread once in a while isn't going to set you back ten steps. *Warning*! This doesn't give your inner fat kid the green light to eat whatever the hell it wants, but you can afford to enjoy some of the things you like because your muscles will eat up the excess calories if you're exercising regularly. Key phrase: exercising regularly.

- **Reduces stress and increase sex drive:** If all of those benefits don't coerce you into changing your exercise habits, I know this one will. Who wants to hump more? Me, me, me! I do. Everyone does! Exercise will get Mr. Willie and Ms. Clyde all happy with blood, which will rev up your sex life in no time! Exercise increases testosterone production, which in turn increases libido. Additionally, its anti-catabolic properties prevent the hormone cortisol from storing fat. Ever wonder why body builders get ripped so damn fast? Hmmm, steroids? After they stop the cycle, they pack on the pounds in the abdominal area because the abundance of testosterone has been subdued. Remember that excuse earlier for not wanting to have sex? I've got a headache! Well, guess what? The female orgasm releases oxytocin, which lowers the main stress hormone Mr. Cortisol. Bada Bing Bada Boom! On top of these amazing effects, regular exercise boosts self-confidence because you finally approve of your body image. What happens next? The pee-pee dance...Bada bing bada BOOM!!!

Exercise increases sex drive, reduces stress, improves sleep, and it also brightens your mood. Hmmm, what just happened here? Adhere to this exercise plan for one month, and your SPI portion of your S.P.I.N.E.™ scores will dramatically improve. The higher the S.P.I.N.E.™ score, the more likely the body will adapt to losing fat. My lovely girlfriend literally just texted me the following: "Today, I was so energetic! Amazing what jaw-dropping sex and great sleep can do!" Maybe I ad-libbed the "amazing jaw dropping" line, but sex and sleep honestly do wonders for de-stressing.

Grandpa H (the nickname for my Dad)
My pops is one spry stud muffin. His ego expands monthly due to compliments he is barraged with. People are astonished to find out his age, "Seventy? No shit, Doc, you look like you're in your 50s!" Of course he exaggerates and tells us that he is still getting hit on by 21 year old blonde sorority sisters, but the compliments are a steady flow. On the contrary, an ex-girlfriend of mine has a father about the same age. He looks like Mr. Burns from the Simpsons. Keeled over, bald, wrinkled skin, and horrible posture due to aches and pain. He smoked and drank for years, and it shows – he looks like he is on the verge of death! What is the difference between the two? My dad knows the value of exercise, while most others do not. They continue to look for quick fixes to undo the years of poor treatment that they have subjected their bodies to. This reminds me, I need to make his ass another workout program. There is nothing like getting a three-minute voicemail from my father saying, "Chrissy boy, the neighbor's dog is an asshole. Gonzaga really sucks. And, thanks for my workout program dickweed. I see how important your father is in your life! Love ya. Pops." Nothing like some good ol' Hitchko lovin'!

Why the VTD is better than the rest
Imagine attaining your dream body by doing less work? Oh boy, here comes the infomercial pitch. Wrong, bucko. This is what happens when you work out smarter and not harder. Most workout programs start off like a New Year's resolution, grandiose and unrealistic. "I'm going to get into the best shape of my life this year!" No, you won't. The average person stops their New Year's Resolution in 19 days — that's two days short of establishing a habit. So close, but you're still fat. What happened? Your goals were too unrealistic. You didn't see the results within a couple of weeks and quit, or you progressed too fast and ended up with an overuse injury. On December 31, you're 100% inactive and overweight, and then on January 2nd (remember on the 1st you're going to be hung-over), you're putting 110% into a new workout program. Where is the proper progression? The body's connective tissue will eventually become inflamed, and you won't be able to continue. Muscles are more vascular, so they will get stronger and faster due to the better quality of nutrients that they receive. The problem lies within the connective tissues themselves (tendons, fascia, and ligaments.) They are avascular (lack blood flow) and do not receive the same amount of nutrients as muscle. The results are the muscles get stronger at the mercy of connective tissue. The muscle belly ends up pulling at the origin and insertion points (connective tissue at beginning and end of a muscle), and it becomes irritated. It's like a game of tug-of-war with two big bullies on one side and the dorky kid on the other. After a while, an injury is inevitable. The body will overrun itself, and you will have to stop working out.

I know this sounds familiar. The average person starts off way too fast and ends up hurt or not achieving his/her long-term goal. If you want to prove me wrong, go to your local track and run a mile. At the sound of the gun, I want you to sprint for the four laps. Ready. Set. Go! Within 300 yards, you're keeled over on the verge of puking. This is exactly what other workout plans are doing to you. They're making false promises like "Lose 10 lbs. in 21 days!" The VTD system progresses your body in a way that it's meant to: nice and slow. I suggest working out three times in week one. Once your body is conditioned to handle more volume and stress (around weeks 4-6), we crank it up! By week six, I challenge you to work out six times, with the bar set at four times per week. A constant worry I hear from beginners is that they want to do more. "My friend Becky is doing *"enter dumb fucking name for an exercise video"* five times a week, so shouldn't I be training that much?" I love your enthusiasm, but you're starting too fast. Save that kick-ass attitude for weeks four and five because that's when you'll need it! Becky is probably going to end up with knee pain in about three weeks and be right back to square one. You on the other hand will be prepared for greater intensities. Before you know it, you'll be pushing through new barriers and sporting looser clothes!

The VTD is better because it's a periodized system that helps you achieve your goals in a realistic, timely, fun, and safe manner by working smarter and not harder. Here's the kicker: VTD is not only addressing exercise and nutrition; it's also tackling your S.P.I.N.E.™. Adjusting all of these aspects of wellness will change your previously shitty habits into better, healthier ones. I will usually add in "perky tits and ass" for the ladies and "ripped abs and constant boners" for guys- you'd be amazed at the response from those selling points!

College and Fat Loss

Think of an exercise program like attending college. It's a four-year program, not just one semester. What do you think would happen if you signed up for 36 units the first semester? You'd be taking 12 classes, you'd go crazy! Strong and steady will get you to the commencement date. In the VTD, I am giving you 9-12 units in the beginning and then progressing you into 15-18 units. By the end, you'll be graduating on time. Graduation is you achieving your fat loss goals. For some, it may be three months, for others it may take longer. The most important take away message is that you'll be graduating and not a drop out as many of us have fallen prey to (not achieving our fat loss goals.) This workout system can be tailored for all types of people. One of the biggest success stories I saw in a client was more than 42 lbs. of scale loss. The end is in sight, but he isn't done yet. He still needs to work hard and eat well. Adhering to the VTD for an additional six months will make him that much closer to his original goal. I wonder how many contestants on weightloss TV shows return home only to slam back on the pounds that they just lost? I bet a lot. It's because no stable system is in place. Where is the education and the teaching? I rarely see episode's where they're teaching the contestants how to properly eat and workout. Its obnoxious militant trainers screaming at them telling them what to do. They're essentially drones following directions with no long-term plan. Not to mention, a lot of these trainers are giving us a bad rep and setting our clients up with unrealistic goals, "I want to lose 29lbs in a week as seen on TV," It doesn't happen that way sweetheart. Mental reminder...make sure to kick a celebrity trainer in the groin next time you meet one. Check. The VTD allows for a lifestyle, not just a quick fix for a few months. Too many programs today start you off with 20+ units, eventually leading to failure. I may come off harsh, but I don't want you to fail. I only want the best for you. Most workout plans suck Bigfoot's balls. Seriously. Imagine Bigfoot's balls in your mouth? All hairy and stinky. Each one would be the size of a baseball. Ewww, that wouldn't be fun! Stick to this system, and you'll be the valedictorian. Don't and you'll be burnt out, smoking crack, turning tricks for pennies on the dollar and sucking Bigfoot's balls. Don't suck Bigfoot's balls people.

Periodization

Periodization is the organized approach to training, which consists of changing the variables during a specific time. VTD is a tailored system for all bodies to succeed. Remember Milo? Yes, you do! How could you forget that awesome picture? Milo implemented periodization without even knowing it. The external weight from his bestie with testies, the Bull, constantly stressed his body to adapt to the new stimulus. As the bull grew, Milo got stronger, and muscular hypertrophy took place (his muscles grew). Now do I believe Milo's story to be true? Probably not, but I do enjoy the idea behind it- stress the body with actual weight and stop lifting pussy weight. If you continue to lift light weight, you're pussy will continue to grow. No one likes big pussies, guys nor girls! The acronym FITT can be used to help with understanding periodization: Frequency, Intensity, Time and Type. Change these four variables every 3-4 weeks, and you'll be on your way to success. I love how books and popular fitness gurus make up their own terms such as "muscle confusion." Marketing agencies must think people aren't smart enough to understand actual scientific terms like periodization, so they dumb it down. Infomercials highlight fat loss programs with phrases like, "Guaranteed results in 30 days." This is extremely unrealistic for the average person. The VTD will allow for safe progression and easy-to-follow workouts until your goals are met. *Spoiler alert! Spoiler alert!* There will be additional books that will help you bust through plateaus and reach new levels of peak fitness through periodization. The VTD workouts will consist of fun and new training variables every workout (this is referred to as undulating periodization). The first day of the workout has you lifting a weight you can appropriately lift for 20 reps. On workout number two, the weight will be increased to an amount you can lift 15 times and so forth.

In the beginning, I want you to lift lighter weights (20 reps) and train the whole body every workout. Half way in, you'll begin decreasing the reps (6-12 rep) and doing split-routines (splitting body parts into segments on different days). At the end, there will be a large increase in intensity, weight, and volume because your body can handle it; it's now in a conditioned state. The proper progression from low to high and light to heavy is exactly what your body needs for proper adaptation. As previously mentioned, too hard and too fast only predestines the body for failure.

There are always anomalies, but for those who follow the VTD as closely to 100% as possible, results will be earned. Just imagine that voice from those Men's Warehouse commercials, "I guarantee it." I have never had someone fail who completely followed my diet and exercise system. The closer you become to functioning naturally by eliminating shitty foods, the more energy and quicker results will be earned. Taking away the chemicals and replacing them with natural ingredients will yield a healthier you. Notice how I said earned? I am giving you the proper tools for amazing results. The ass-kicking hard work is up to you. Now, let me teach you the essentials of resistance training.

Weight Lifting 101

There are seven main muscle groups that we use in the gym (large to small): legs, back, chest, shoulders, triceps, biceps, and core. Core represents the abs, oblique's, and lower back. The core works in synergy. If you want to workout smarter, stop wasting time, and follow these rules for maximal fat loss:

1. Work larger muscles first, and progress into smaller ones: legs before chest and chest before shoulders.
2. Multi-jointed before single-jointed exercises. Step ups before leg extensions. Push-ups before chest flies. Chin-ups before bicep curls. Planks before abs. Then again, why are you isolating your abs?

By implementing methods one and two, your heart will be forced to work harder. This releases more powerful hormones and burns calories more efficiently. Not sold? Drop down and do 25 crunches. Now, check your pulse for 10 seconds by locating your radial artery (pulse below your thumb where your wrist and hand meet). If you multiply that number by six, that's how many beats per minute your heart is pumping. Now, record that number here_____.

Next, I want you to do 25 body weight squats into a chair and follow suit. Record that number here_____.

Now, I want you to take a topless photo and send it to my address here_____. Did that work? Dammit! It was worth a try.

Which exercise produced a higher heart rate response? Body weight squats just ninja-kicked crunches right in the fucking jugular - Hiyaaaa! I just did this example personally, and my numbers were 78 for crunches and 120 for squats. That means my heart worked an extra 75 beats per minute compared to the crunches. Did you catch it? That was a test to see if you're actually thinking while reading because my heart was only working an extra 42 beats per minute, gotcha! What does this mean? Endless crunches won't do shit for your six pack. Nor will tricep extensions or bicep curls do shit for defined arms. We need to burn away the layer of fat, which means burning more calories. Squats and/or multi-jointed exercises will induce a higher heart rate response, which in turn will burn more calories. Push-ups would be far superior to tricep extensions for nice arms, as would chin-ups instead of bicep curls. The abduction machines are a joke, so no mas! If you want to settle for mediocrity, then keep on doing those dumb-ass exercises. The answers to the beckoning cry, "I have tried everything!" lie within the VTD workout system.

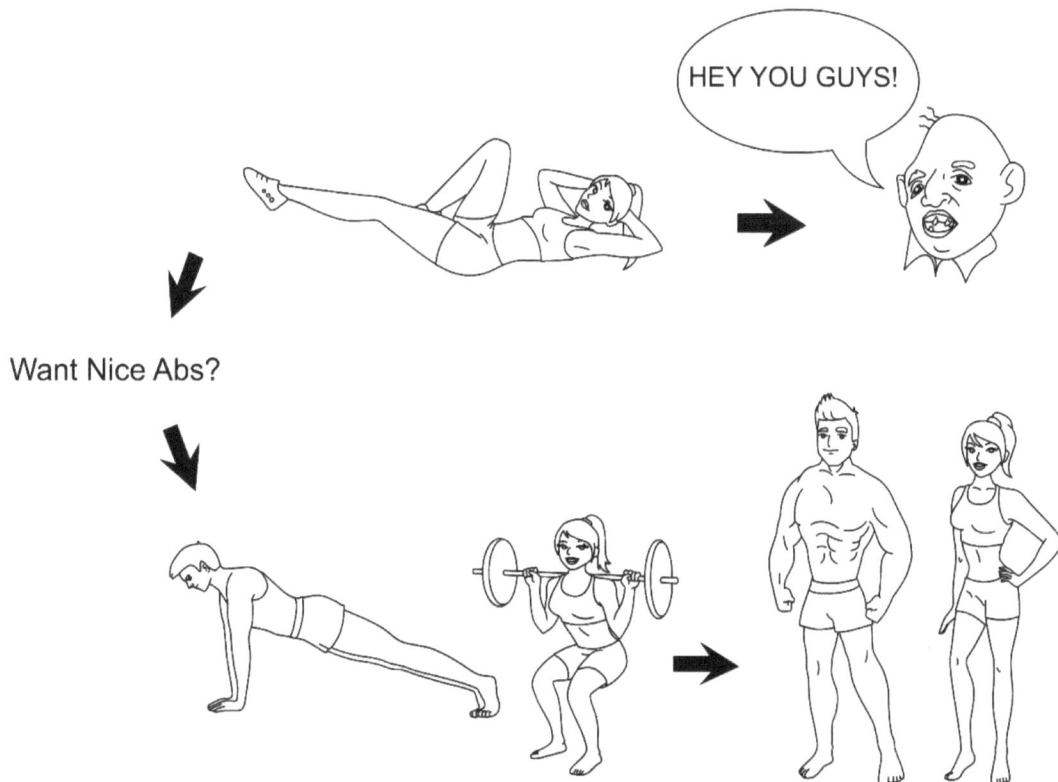

HEY YOU GUYS!

Want Nice Abs?

That's Sloth in the upper right hand corner. Come on peeps, remember *Goonies??*
While examining Milo and his success, we can adopt his resiliency for perfection by mimicking his behavior of constant overload by way of repetitions. For optimal results, resistance training should be performed a minimum of four times a week. Aim for targeting each of the seven muscle groups at least twice per week.

Energy Tanks

Every cell in the body uses Adenosine Triphosphate (ATP) as the chief energy source for movement. We can create ATP from sugar (glucose), fat, and protein. Our brain's primary fuel source is sugar. When our blood sugar levels run low, we can get more from the stored form of energy in our liver and muscles, which is called glycogen. Think of glucose as water and glycogen as ice cubes in the freezer. Fat yields more *ATP than the other substrates, but before we can use fat, we have to burn off the sugar first. When our muscles perform work, muscle glycogen is depleted. Using resistance for exercise (especially multi-joint before single and large before small), will deplete sugar faster than any other type of exercise (cardio included). *One triglyceride (fat) molecule yields over 460 ATP molecules, whereas one glucose molecule yields just a little over 30.

When you go for a run, the intensity isn't as high; therefore, muscle glycogen will take longer to deplete. A half-hour run won't burn much fat. The faster we deplete the sugar, the quicker we can get into using fat as the primary fuel source. Who wants to burn fat doing your workouts? Everyone! Weight training is the answer. If you want to perform cardio, do it after weight training. No more cardio by itself unless it's fasted or HIIT. These two exceptions get into the fat storage a lot faster because your sugar tank is empty (fasted), and/or the intensity is higher (HIIT). Adhering to methods 1-2 and the VTD system will deplete muscle glycogen faster. Afterward, performing cardio will maximize the fat burning. You're welcome. You are now working out smarter instead of harder.
 To my astonishment, the average person doesn't have the slightest clue about what muscles are being engaged during a workout program. It's not anyones fault; most people haven't been taught properly. Let Senior Christobol teach you the basics. Here are some cliff notes for lifting weights:

- Push forward = Chest and Triceps
- Push overhead = Shoulders and Triceps
- Pull up / down = Back and Biceps

Specific exercises for each muscle:

- Chest = Push-Up, Bench Press, and Chest Fly
- Back = Pull-Up, Lat Pull-Down, and Dumbbell Row
- Shoulders = Military Press, Arnold press, Upright Row, and Rotating T's
- Legs = Squats, Lunges, RDLs, Leg Press & Jumps

Keep in mind anytime that you alter your grip during an exercise, the emphasis on the muscles may change. Take the push-up with a standard hand position, for example. When you press away from the ground, the muscles engaged are the chest and triceps. Now, if you move your hands 12 inches (within a finger's distance apart, aka diamond push-up) the chest and triceps are still being recruited, but the triceps become the main emphasis due to the greater extension that is taking place at the elbow. Here are some examples of alternating grips, which will put a different emphasis on another muscle.

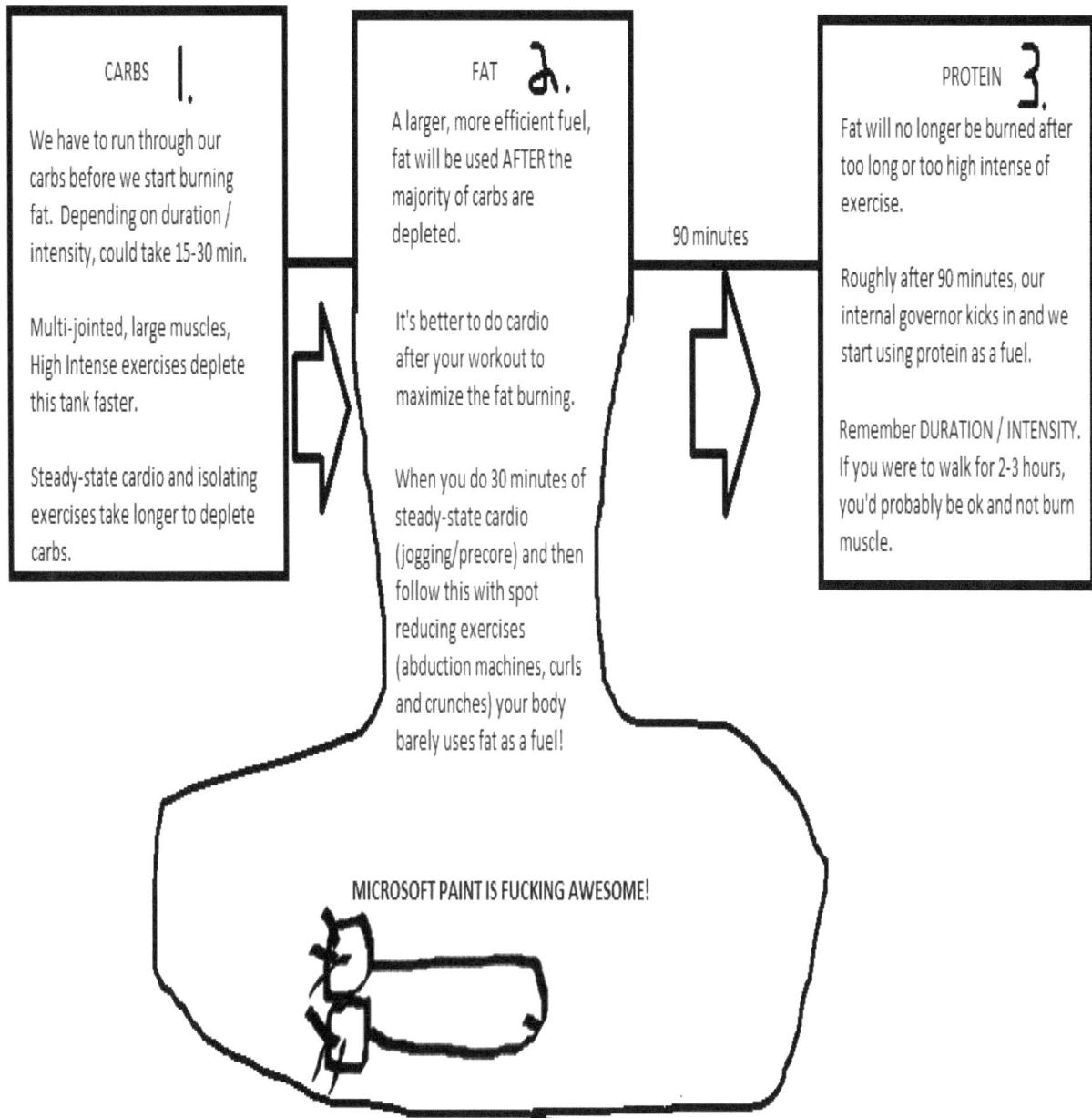

CARBS 1.

We have to run through our carbs before we start burning fat. Depending on duration / intensity, could take 15-30 min.

Multi-jointed, large muscles, High Intense exercises deplete this tank faster.

Steady-state cardio and isolating exercises take longer to deplete carbs.

FAT 2.

A larger, more efficient fuel, fat will be used AFTER the majority of carbs are depleted.

It's better to do cardio after your workout to maximize the fat burning.

When you do 30 minutes of steady-state cardio (jogging/precore) and then follow this with spot reducing exercises (abduction machines, curls and crunches) your body barely uses fat as a fuel!

90 minutes

PROTEIN 3.

Fat will no longer be burned after too long or too high intense of exercise.

Roughly after 90 minutes, our internal governor kicks in and we start using protein as a fuel.

Remember DURATION / INTENSITY. If you were to walk for 2-3 hours, you'd probably be ok and not burn muscle.

MICROSOFT PAINT IS FUCKING AWESOME!

Pull-Up:
Shoulder width apart = Back and biceps.
Alter the grip so your palms are facing your face (chin up), and then the emphasis goes to your biceps.
Alter the grip so your hands are extremely wide, and then the emphasis goes to mainly your back.

Squat:
Shoulder width apart = Glutes, quads, and hamstrings
Alter your stance and move your legs further away (Plie squat), and then the glutes become the main emphasis.
Front squat (the barbell or kettle bell is in front of the chest), and then the quads become the main emphasis.

Back:

Cable row (neutral grip) = Back and Biceps with the emphasis being mainly your back. Alter the grip to a wide grip, and then the emphasis goes to your posterior deltoids.

Shoulders:
Military Press = Anterior & medial deltoid and triceps
Alter the motion by adding a twist (Arnold press), and now all three parts of the deltoid are engaged.

All of these exercises are multi-jointed. You'll notice that the biceps and triceps are engaged quite a lot, so why do we need to isolate them? We really don't need to unless you are trying to build them excessively, i.e. body builders. Don't get me started on bodybuilders.

If you want nice arms, do more pushing (push-up & bench press), pulling (pull-ups, rows, and pull-downs), and pushing overhead exercises (military and Arnold presses). If you are uncertain, go back to the previous crunch versus lunge exercise and perform the same demo for bicep curls versus lat pull-downs.

Rep and Rest Ranges
You probably constantly see the following in magazines: 3 x 10, 2 x 15 or 5 x 5. What the fuck is this, high school math? No, no, no. Relax: These numbers represent how many repetitions and sets you will be doing. The first number tells you how many cycles you will be performing that exercise or circuit for. The second number corresponds with how many times you will be performing the exercise. Bench Press 5 x 15 translates into 15 repetitions for five cycles. Each cycle is separated by rest. Longer rest periods are needed for heavier loads. The rule of thumb is the following:

- Weight that can be lifted more than 12 times, you should rest less than one minute.
- Weight that can be lifted between 6-12 times, you should rest between 1-3 minutes.
- Maximal and powerful/explosive weights that can be lifted between 1-5 times, you should rest between 3-5 minutes.

Remember that these are guidelines, and if you ever need longer rest periods, go for it! At any point if you begin to feel lightheaded or dizzy, take a longer rest breaks. There may be times during the high intensity workouts that these symptoms may arise, especially with low carbs. Don't freak out and have a panic attack. This happens all the time, trust me, and you aren't going to die. Your blood sugar levels have significantly dropped, and you need to get sugar to your brain ASAP! This is why I suggest always carrying a banana, Cliff Bar, or Gatorade with you just in case of an emergency. I have had students and clients push too hard during high intensity interval days, and this situation occurs. They become extremely lightheaded and feel like they are going to pass out or throw up. Some even do throw up and pass out. This exercise-induced barf session is usually caused by the tornado of hormones that have just been released (endorphins and growth hormone). Additionally, it could be from dehydration, de-conditioning, and poor nutrition. Just make sure to get some sugar into your system and allow 15 minutes for it to go away. The worse thing that you can do is worry; this will just exacerbate the symptoms. One time I did sprints up these hills and was a little too gung-ho. About 15 minutes into the workout, I started to lose my vision, and I definitely freaked the fuck out! I called my parents' house for some coddling, but my dad answered. He started laughing and said, "Yep, you're gonna die!" That definitely didn't help. Luckily, my mom stole the phone away, and her soothing voice made everything all right. I'm such a pussy.

On that topic, another note to mention is pre-workout drinks. These supplements have a shit ton of caffeine and chemicals, but they do give you crazy amounts of energy. I urge caution with these supplements. I don't suggest taking any, but if you do, just be aware. The dizziness factor is definitely more prone to happen after taking 1-2 servings of your favorite pre-workout drink. If you are really lagging and need a pick-me-up, opt for a cup of black coffee instead. Less chemicals and way better for you in the long run! I literally just had a student stop her workout because she felt ill from experimenting with one of the newer name brands of pre workout drinks. Question. Where do supplement companies come up with the fucked up names for their brands? If I were to name a supplement, I would name it "Achillobator's Ripped Cock Fuel". Achillobator was a badass dinosaur similar to a raptor. Its name comes from the Greek hero Achilles and also the Mongolian root for "warrior." The rest of my supplement name speaks for itself.

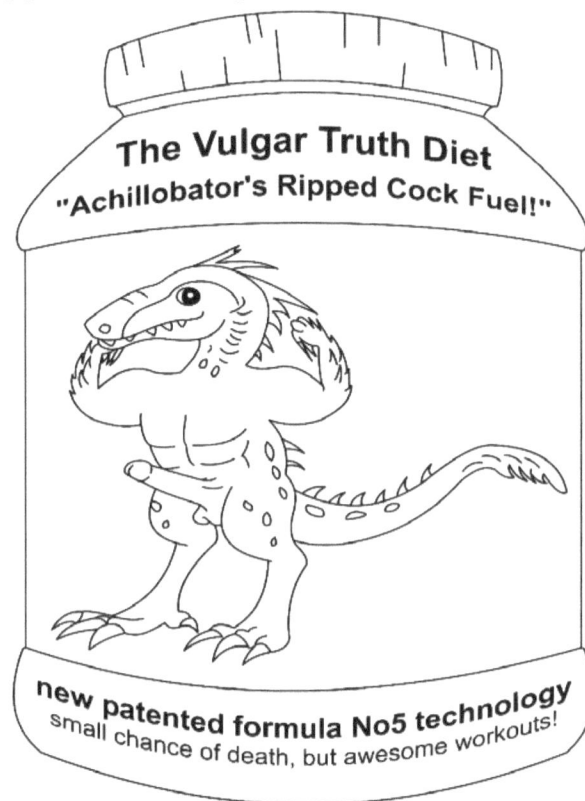

Sorry supplement companies, but you're benefiting from people's ignorance. The anecdotal evidence is superb, but what about the science? The majority of pre-workout products are big piles of placebo shit carrying enough unknown chemicals to probably make your dick fall off. A rule of thumb that I abide by: if you can't pronounce an ingredient on the bottle, then stay the fuck away from it!

Adaptations
I continually emphasize that you stick with any system for a minimum of 30 days. The behavioral and psychological aspects of S.P.I.N.E.™ are the main reasons. There is another reason, to allow for neural adaptations. During the first couple of months of any resistance training program, the main adaptations that take place are neurological, aka your brain learning how to communicate effectively with your muscles. Neurological communication is the equivalent of boot camp. Not the fru-fru bootcamps where you go and workout outside. I am talking about military bootcamps. These 4-6 week periods mentally prepare you for war. Don't expect large amounts of

fat loss and/or muscle growth, because your body's main goal is to learn how to communicate efficiently. After bootcamp, your body is conditioned and ready to handle more.

How many times have you stopped a workout program within a month because you weren't seeing results? "Well, I saw contestants on a TV show lose 21lbs. in a week, and I know that's real because the trainer cried." You need to understand that magazines, infomercials, and the media fabricate the truth. These are not typical results, and they are augmented. Imagine going to a clinic with personal trainers, doctors, and registered dietitians who monitor your workouts and diets hourly. Extreme weight loss will occur because the envelope can be pushed. If this scenario doesn't sound like your life, don't expect the same results. Don't throw a hissy fit; results will be earned through VTD, but it takes time. Losing 2-5 pounds of fat during the first month is awesome work, but remember you won't be weighing yourself until the end of the system. Ninety days isn't that long; give it a shot and look back and see for yourself.

Muscle Fiber Types
To simplify, there are two types of muscle fibers: slow twitch (type I) and fast twitch (type II). The former are deep muscles that stabilize the body as seen in the core, rotator cuff, and spinal column. They are able to work for longer periods of time, but they lack the ability to grow and produce high amounts of force as seen in their fast twitch counterparts.

Fast twitch muscle are primarily recruited in the following situations: maximal force production, max velocities, and during times of complete exhaustion. Type II muscles are very powerful, lie at the surface of the body, and are much larger, i.e. quads, hamstrings, glutes, chest, and back. My goal throughout the VTD is to teach your body how to move properly in the first 4-6 weeks. After this, I want you lifting heavier weights and moving faster to maximize results. The more muscle that you put on, the more your body becomes metabolically efficient (better at burning fat).
Who wants to turn into a badass fat-burning machine? Everyone does! I know half of you girls reading up to this point just slightly soiled your sexy thong underwear because I said lifting "heavier weights." I'll say it again; you won't get big and bulky. In actuality, your body will shrink up and get smaller. No shit? Muscle is more active (requires more calories to maintain itself), so the more of it that you have, the tighter you will become. Think of it like this: Imagine an empty tissue box. Place the tissue box inside of a small duffle bag. If you are actually performing this demonstration, there will be a decent amount of space between the box and the bag. That space represents fat. When we lift heavier weights, we begin to fill the tissue box with tissues. Additionally, the space between the bag and the box will be compressed, as if the air has been sucked out of it. After three months of the VTD, your tissue box will be full and the bag will be compressed around it like a tightly packed Christmas present. Has the box grown? No, not at all. The total package actually shrunk a shitload! The box, aka your muscle, will become denser. Strong is the new skinny, ladies, so pick up the heavier weights and become superior. If you continue to lift those light weights, you are settling for inferiority and a soft body.

For the males, your tissue box will get bigger because you have a lot more testosterone than females do. This is one of the unfair advantages that we have. If you train properly, you are primed to pack on the muscle in a shorter timeframe than women. Remember, knowledge is power. Educating yourself on how the body works is going to make the experience of weight training more valuable. Ignorance isn't always bliss. Knowing which muscles are working during every exercise makes it that much more enjoyable. Turn on that thinker and become thirsty for knowledge. Working out will be fun during the VTD! The amount of filth flooding the newsstands makes it hard to understand what is valid and what is hogwash. When it doubt, human anatomy and physiology is rarely wrong. If a trainer doesn't know much about human anatomy, how can they seriously help you achieve your fitness-related goals?

What Makes Someone an Expert?

"My name is Tooloff, and I used to weigh 300lbs., and I lost 150lbs. in a year."

Awesome story, Mr. Tooloff, but that success story doesn't make you an expert in the field of exercise. Our industry is saturated with people exactly like this. They had success losing weight, so they go online, get certified, and then call themselves experts. I had a friend beat cancer. Does that make him an expert in Oncology? Does he have the right to start up his own cancer-fighting clinic? No way for fucks sake! You may listen to some best practices, but you wouldn't pay money for the advice over going to a doctor who specializes in Oncology. He doesn't know the science behind what he just beat. Doctors do; that's why they're experts.

I am going to look at four true fitness experts in the industry. I would love to compare them to some recognized "experts" in the general public's eye, but my lawyer said I could get sued up the ying-yang, so I'll keep it PC- fucking law suits, ruining all the fun.

- **<u>Len Kravitz (not the singer)</u>**, Ph.D. - Health Promotion and Exercise Science, University of New Mexico
- 1999 to present: Associate Professor of Exercise Science, The University of New Mexico
- Honors/Awards:
  - Canadian Fitness Specialty Presenter of the Years, 2009 and 2006.
  - Senior Exercise Physiologist, IDEA - The Health and Fitness Source (Media Spokesperson), 2003 - 2005
  - Lifetime Achievement, ECA World Fitness Association, 2003
  - Researcher of the Year, The University of Mississippi, College of Education, 1999

His website may be old fashioned, but this is one badass dude!

- **<u>William J. Kraemer</u>**, Ph.D. - Physiology and Biochemistry, University of Wyoming
- Professor of Kinesiology, Physiology, Neurobiology & Medicine at The University of Connecticut - Present

  Honors/Awards:
- 2002 - Educator of the Year, National Strength and Conditioning Association (NSCA)
- 1994 - Lifetime Achievement Award from National Strength and Conditioning Association
- 1992 - Outstanding Sport Scientist Award from National Strength and Conditioning Association

To summarize, Dr. Kraemer is the Michael Jordan of fitness. He is the Godfather. I got an "A" in a class at Chico because I name-dropped him. Anytime I talk to him, I get butterflies like a high school boy, it's cute so shut up.

- **<u>Dr. Mike Clark</u>** - DPT, MS, CPT. Doctor of physical therapy from Rocky Mountain University. Clark is the chief executive officer of the National Academy of Sports Medicine (NASM).
- Creator of NASM's exclusive Optimum Performance Training™ (OPT) model used by thousands of health and fitness professionals worldwide.
- Recognized as one of the top physical therapists in the nation.

To summarize, Dr. Clark has revolutionized personal training, making it a safer place by putting more educated trainers on the market.

- **Alwyn Cosgrove** - Degree in Sports Performance at West Lothian College, then progressed on to receiving an honors degree in Sports Science from Chester College, the University of Liverpool.
- He is the architect behind the programming for amazing books such as: *The New Rules of Weight Lifting,* and the book for women.
- One of the most successful fitness facilities in the country www.results-fitness.com.

To summarize, he is from England so the school systems are different; he probably went to "university" and drank tea with crumpets, but nonetheless, still a BADASS. He is one of the most respected trainers, educators and presenters in the fitness community.

How to become a personal trainer
The easiest way to become a certified personal trainer is by ordering the online material, make sure you're older than 18, have a high school diploma or GED, and then sign up and pass the 100 – 150 question test. Within a few weeks you're on the right path to becoming one of the leading health and wellness experts in the world. Good God almighty, Shrek could pass these exams! If you enjoy your experience at the dentist, can you become a licensed dentist in a few days? I don't think so. There are more requirements for apprenticeships or trade schools to become a mechanic or master crafts-worker in welding. It literally takes more education for someone to operate heavy machinery over operating a human life. Something is wrong here people! I am not saying that trainers need to have Ph.Ds, but they should have something a little more detailed than a take-home test. That's why I love teaching at a school that has a combination of 500 hours of anatomy, physiology, nutrition, and bio-mechanics- that's a damn good starting point for becoming a qualified trainer.

I applaud any individual who inspires people to get off their fat asses and exercise. Whether a DVD, infomercial gadget, TV show, unqualified trainer or website, these people are trying to help others live a better life, so great job! Is there a nice, warm place in my heart somewhere? Maybe, but I am still a prick when it comes to credentials and qualifications. We need to second guess who we are venerating as fitness professionals. Many people are being overlook (as scene in the list above), so I want to thank you all for your awesome scientific breakthroughs in science.

Educate yourself properly before you start teaching to the masses about exercise. Just because you're genetically blessed it doesn't give you the right to start preaching. I could give a rat's ass about how ripped you are or how awesome your ass looks in those tiny shorts. You need to teach people properly and stop making the fitness industry toxic. There is something poisonous about this industry that reeks of cat piss. There needs to be uniformity and structure, and not the kind where you can consider yourself a fitness guru or professional because you lost a shit ton of weigh. This doesn't qualify you with a deep understanding of the human body.

Just remember this: a good personal trainer understands the human body, most personal trainers today understand their bodies. That's what us nerds refer to as anecdotal evidence. Until you understand the human body, don't talk to me. Go to school and get a real education.

Hiring a Personal Trainer
For some, following a program individually may not be realistic. I suggest finding a qualified personal trainer. Having that extra motivation is what many people need in order to reach their fitness goals. I have been in the industry for many years and have been exposed to a handful of quality trainers. The vast majority speaks confidently as if they know what they're talking about, but they don't know shit from Shinola! Aesthetically, they may look amazing with broad shoulders, wide back muscles, ripped abs, and defined serratus muscles (muscles just below the arm pit and chest). Don't be fooled; they could just be disciplined or have amazing genetics. Don't be vulnerable. Do yourself a favor and research a trainer you're interested in. If a trainer insists on training you the first session before any type of assessment, be very hesitant. A physical activity readiness questionnaire (PAR-Q) and proper assessment should be the first thing reviewed. During this time, your blood pressure, circumference measurements, and body fat percentage will be taken. A detailed conversation about your goals, medical history, other medical conditions, and injuries should also be reviewed in depth. Doctors don't start surgery without asking questions, do they? Granted we are not doctors, but trainers should take the time to learn your body and listen to what your goals are. Why do trainers have a bad name? Too many times they blabber on too much or push clients too hard and fast, which may cause injuries and even death.

When trying to find a quality trainer, experience doesn't mean jack! If your trainer has a web page with a bunch of shirtless pictures, move on to the next one. I would be lying if I said I have never taken a picture with my shirt off; sex sells, and people are attracted to the human form. But, there is a difference between classy and showing off. A picture that says, "Look at my body. I am better than you," says the trainer is conceded with an IQ equivalent to a rock. Or, just because you lost 60 lbs. on a TV show, it doesn't mean you know how to train other people. You understand your body, not the next person's.

Qualified personal trainers are like diamonds in a ruff. If my words offend you, get over yourself; you're probably a shitty trainer. If you're reading this and laughing along, you completely understand that the training industry is infiltrated with diarrhea. There needs to be some sort of regulating body like the *United States Medical Licensing Examination* (*USMLE*). I know there are Acts that are "trying" to be pushed through Congress that uniformly qualify the industry as a whole. Well, hurry the fuck up! How many people have been injured from working with a trainer? Too many to count. Bottom line: would you go to a doctor just because he/she is good looking?

When it comes to fitness, you need to find a trainer who has legitimate credentials. A degree in Fine Arts or a weekend workshop does not qualify. Look for some of the following: BS or MS in Kinesiology/Exercise Physiology or a diploma from a personal training school such as the National Personal Training Institute (NPTI) or Bryan University (which is online, but still very good). If the trainer has a biography, look for the following certifications (in this order): CSCS, NSCA, ACSM, NASM or a personal training school like NPTI. In my opinion, they are the top certifications in the industry. Don't be afraid to ask for references either. Make sure they have helped similar people achieve their goals.

Personal Trainer Disclaimer!
Sorry for beating the shit out of a dead horse, but I want to make it clear that I'm not bashing ALL trainers. There're some trainers who have done the self-taught route and are helping people live healthier lives. I'm just encouraging you to challenge any trainer you work with. Ask them about

anatomy. Do they know the names of the rotator cuff muscles (supraspinatus, infraspinatus, teres minor and subscapularis)? If you want to be a complete prick like me, make them name all 17 muscles that attach around the shoulder. If they can't, I fart as loud as I can and walk away. Ask for references. How long did it take them to become a trainer? Did they spend a solid 30-60 minutes reviewing your goals, exercise and health history before they started training you? There are many "YouTube trainers" out there showcasing the trendiest exercises, but don't know shit about the human body or how it actually works. If you're looking for the best, trainers with CSCS (certified strength and conditioning specialist) are USUALLY superior. The CSCS exam requires infinite knowledge in anatomy, biomechanics and physiology- not to mention, a college degree.

The Workout:
High intense workouts or classes with a lot of jumping and complex movements are great programs for CONDITIONED individuals. I concede that these types of workouts are truly difficult and can potentially yield amazing results, but what happens to those who push too hard and get injured from overtraining or improper form? Tough! You won't be mentioned in the infomercial testimonials because you're just a big pussy! As I said, these workouts are tough as elephant manure; just understand that they aren't for everyone. The VTD differs from the rest because this workout is tailored for you. Yes, you, reading this book right now. Whether you're a beginner, desk jockey, nurse, student, or banker, the VTD will work for you.

I will progress you in a scientific manner, which will allow for your ligaments and tendons to properly adapt and not burn out from some sort of "itis." Follow the workouts as close to 100% as you can, and you will see results. Without further ado, here is the *VTD Fat Loss* workout system.

MONTH-AT-A-GLANCE BLANK CALENDAR

MONTH _____

Sunday	Monday	Tuesday	Wednesday	Thursday	Friday	Saturday

FOR MORE INFORMATION ON PROPER FORM, PLEASE GO TO WWW.SHOWUPFITNESS.COM

Warm up for weeks 1-3
- Knee Pulls (pull knee to chest)
- Ankle Pulls (pull ankle to butt)
- Open ups (bring knee to chest and then rotate / "open up" to the side
- Step-ups with kick back (10 per side)
- Modified Jumps (50%)
- Plank

Week 1: Full Body

Leg Press or Squats with a press (See image below)

Bench Press* if you cannot use the bar (45lbs) use a chest machine or dumbbells as seen in the images below.

Cable Row (Ideally wide grip) (See image below)

Military Press (See image below)

Accessory muscles – Floor Bridges (See image below)

Walk for 20-30 minutes at 3-3.5mph @ incline of 5-10

- 3 total sets per exercise: 20 reps (increase the weight / rest for 1 minute), 15 reps (increase the weight / rest for 1 minute), 12 reps (move onto next exercise)
- Workout 3 non-consecutive days.
- Rest 1 minute (basically the time it takes to add weights and count to 30) OR if with a workout partner, the time it takes for them to complete their set.
- Tempo for each repetition will be 1x1 (1 second down and 1 second up)

Squats (add in a military press to maximize caloric expenditure):

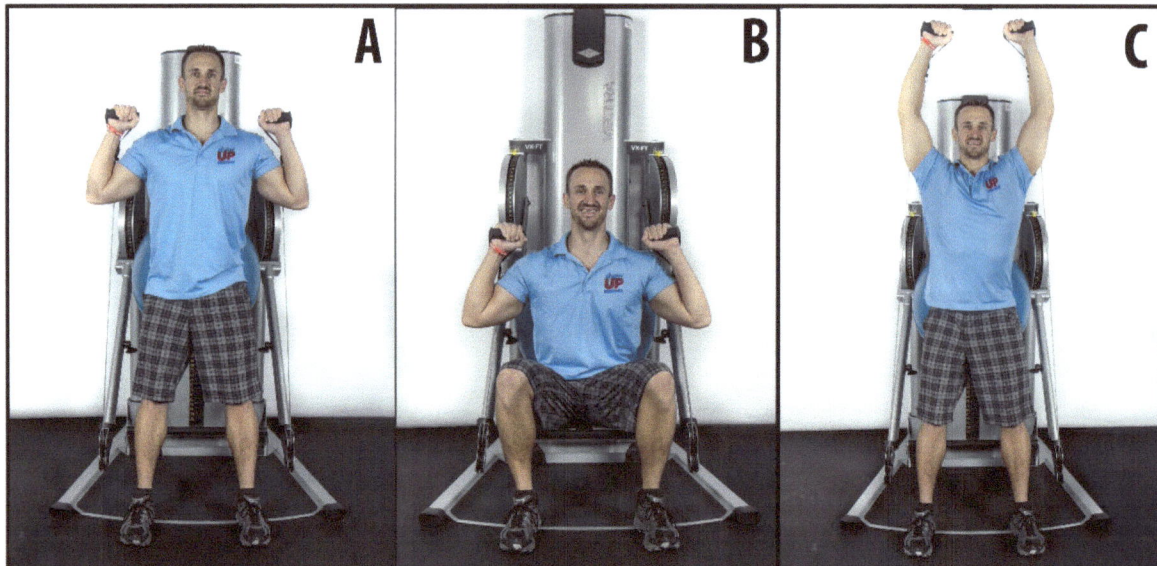

A) If you have a machine like this, place a stability ball behind you. If not, use a stability ball on a hard surface (be careful of performing this exercise on a mirror; don't want 7 years of bad luck!)
B) Squat down so your femur bone (thighs) go below parallel to the ground. See how my scrumptious ass is below my kneecaps? By doing this (going below 90 degrees), you're glutes will be engaged a lot more.
C) As you come up, press your knees out (external rotation) and drive through your heels. If you are performing the press, press the weights over your head to finish repetition number 1.

Bench Press / Incline Press (as seen in this picture):

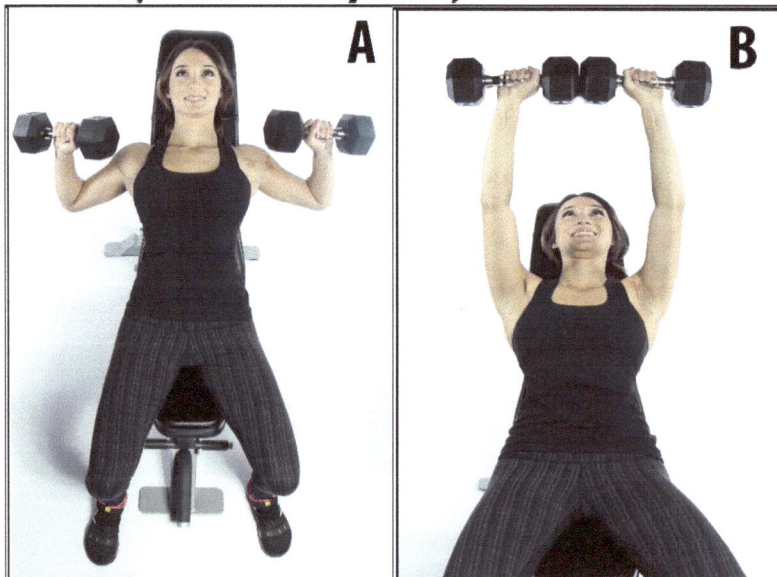

A) Start by bringing the dumbbells to your shoulders
B) Press the weights up and over your chest (upper chest for incline as seen here.) When you lower the weights back down, it's ok to lower your arms below parallel, almost as if the ends of the weights were going to touch the front part of your shoulders. A big misconception is stopping at 90 degrees- that's horseshit! At the end, slightly touch the weights together. *Be cautious* if the weights are metal. Small chunks of metal may fall into your eyes if you bang the weights too hard together. If you have shoulder pain, avoid the incline and any exercise that causes pain.

Cable Row:

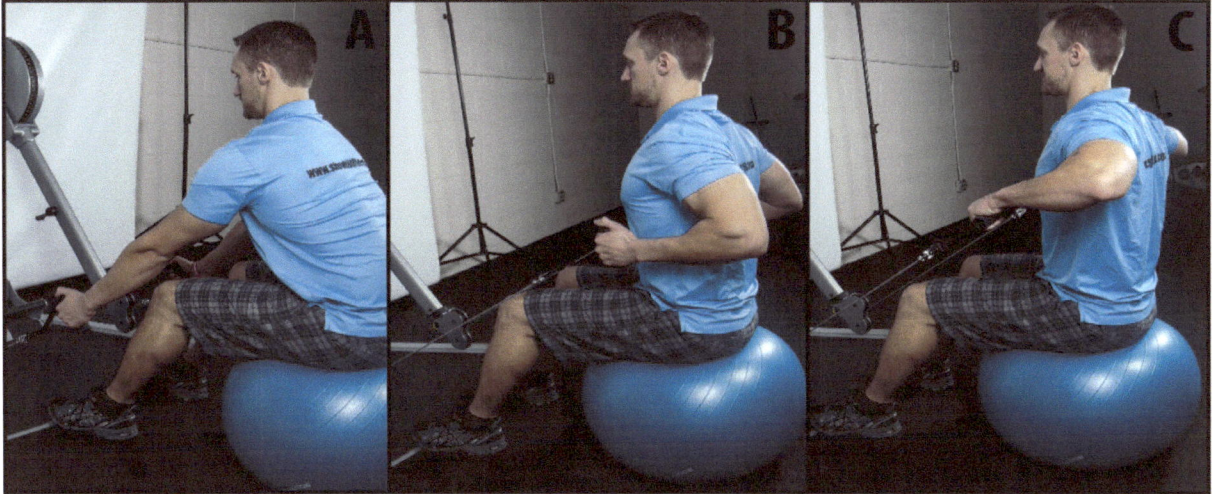

A) Fully extend your arms and unlock your shoulder blades (fully protract).
B) Pull the bar / handles to the side of your stomach as if you were starting a lawn mower.
C) To engage the weaker poster deltoid muscles, rotate your hands so your knuckles are pointing up (pronation).

Military Press:

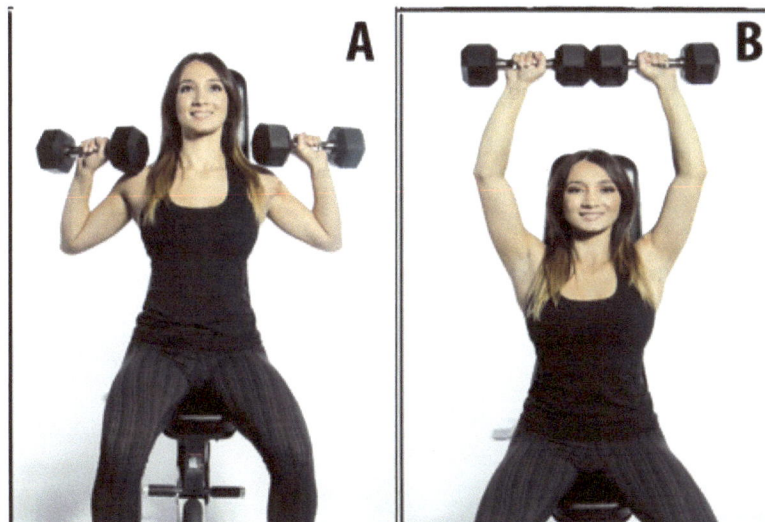

A) Start by bringing the dumbbells to your shoulders (sometimes it helps when the weights become too heavy to begin with the dumbbells on your knees and bounce them up to your shoulders.)
B) Press the weights above your head and slightly touch the dumbbells together. When you lower the weights, bring the dumbbells to the side of your shoulders. As with the bench press, it is OK to lower the weight so your arms go below parallel.

Floor Bridges:

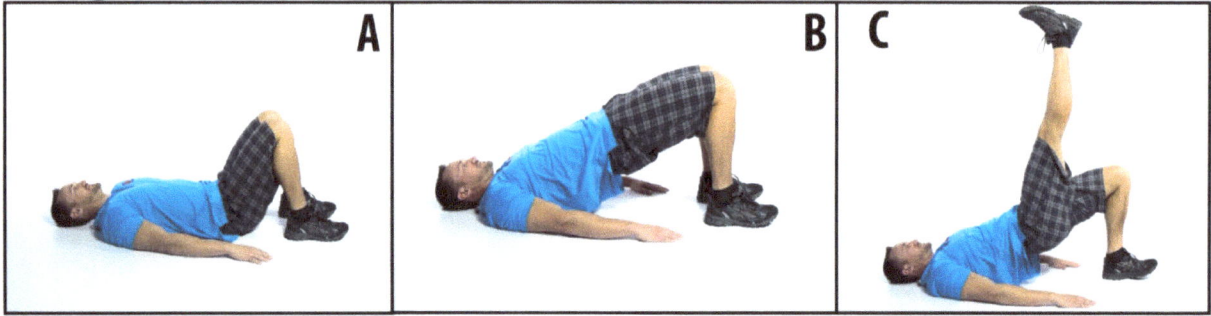

A) Start with your hands by your side and feet facing forward. Your heels should be under your knees.

B) Slowly lift (extend) your glutes off the floor until your body is perpendicular to the floor. Hold at the top for 5 seconds. Make sure to pinch your ass cheeks together as if there was a magical $5,000 dollar bill between them. In a controlled manner, lower your glutes back to A.

C) Progression: Use one leg C or BOSU ball, pulse at the bottom for 10 reps or perform a hip thrust.

Week 2: Full Body (*Tempo 3:1:3)

Step up with a Curl
Bench Press
Lat Pull-down
Arnold Press

Accessory muscles- Hip Thrusters

Walk for 20-30 minutes at 3-3.5mph @ incline of 5-10

- 1 day of fasted cardio (30-60 minute walk/run) OR AM workout
- Workout 3 non-consecutive days with weights + 1 day of cardio OR 1 AM workout
- 3 total sets per exercise: 12 reps (increase the weight / rest for 1 minute), 10 reps (increase the weight / rest for 1 minute), stay at same weight for 10 reps (move onto next exercise)
- *Tempo for each repetition will be 3 x 1 x 3 (3 seconds down, 1 second pause, 3 seconds up) * note that the weight will probably be the same, if not LOWER than the week before due to the timing aspect.

Step Up with a bicep curl:

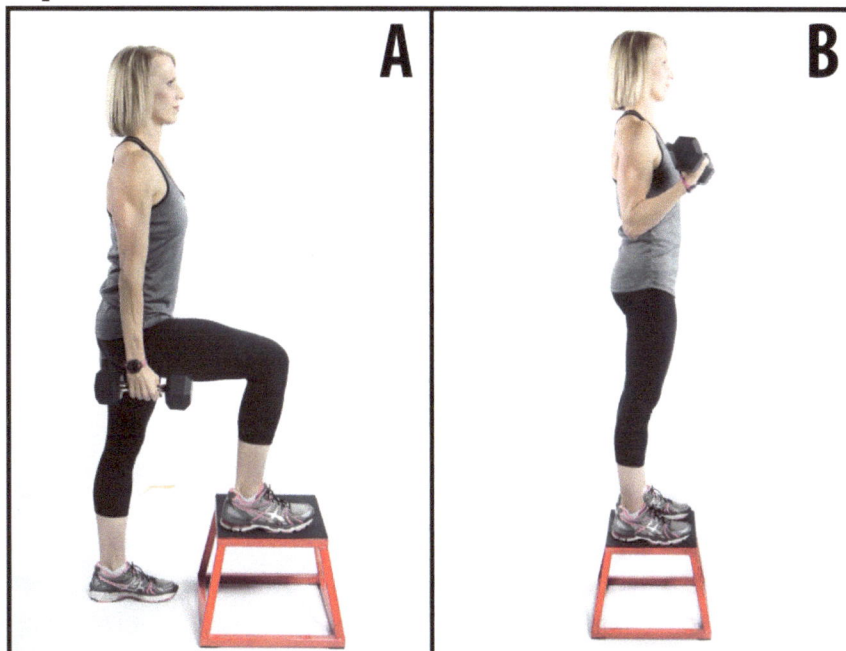

A) Start by finding a chair, step, bench or plyo box as seen in this image. The higher the box, the more the glutes are engaged.

B) Step up onto the box while curling at the same time. Make sure not to cheat and push too much off the trailing leg. Step down with the same leg and repeat 12 times then switch legs.

Lat pull-down:

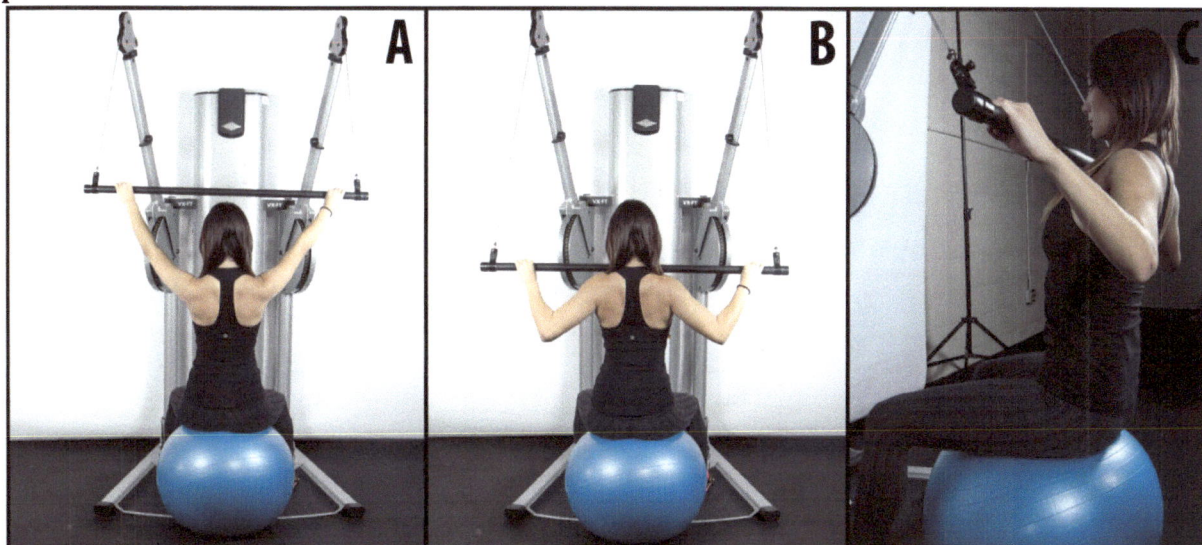

A) Begin with your hands 6-12 inches beyond shoulder width apart. The wider the grip, the more the lats are engaged. The closer the grip the more the biceps are engaged- just image a chin-up!

B) Pull the bar down to the upper part of the chest- slightly below the clavicle C). *Be careful* don't pull TO the clavicle, as the collar bone is the most broken bone in the human body.

Arnold Press:

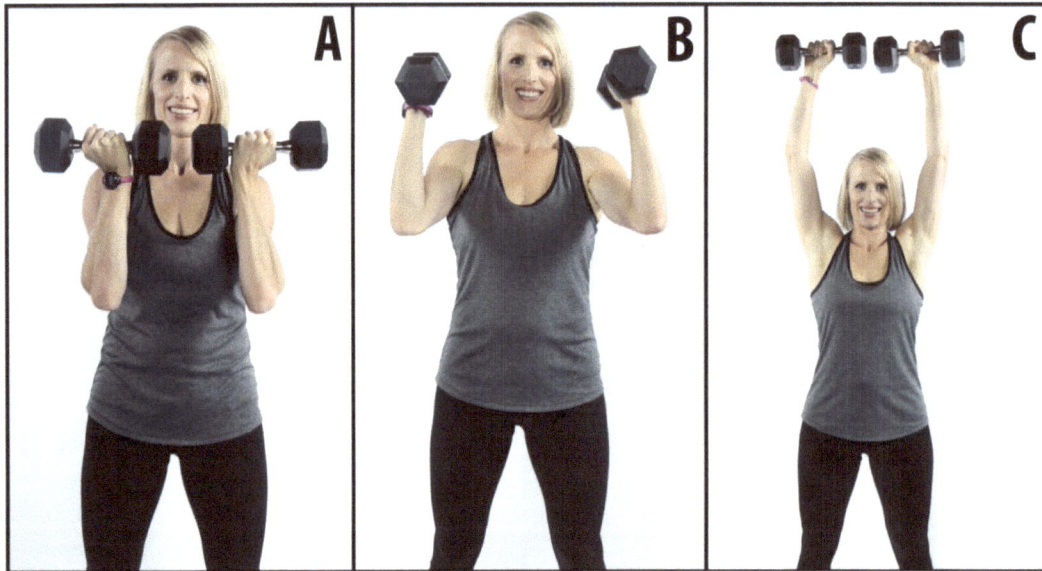

A) Named after the GOVNA himself, the Arnold press is arguably one of the better shoulder exercises because it recruits all three heads of the deltoids. Begin with your palms facing forward.

B) Twist your hands away from one another while keeping them as close to the face as possible.

C) Finish the exercise by pressing overhead as seen in the regular military press. *Be cautious,* due to the twisting aspect of this exercise, the weight used should be LOWER than that of the military press.

Hip Thrusters:

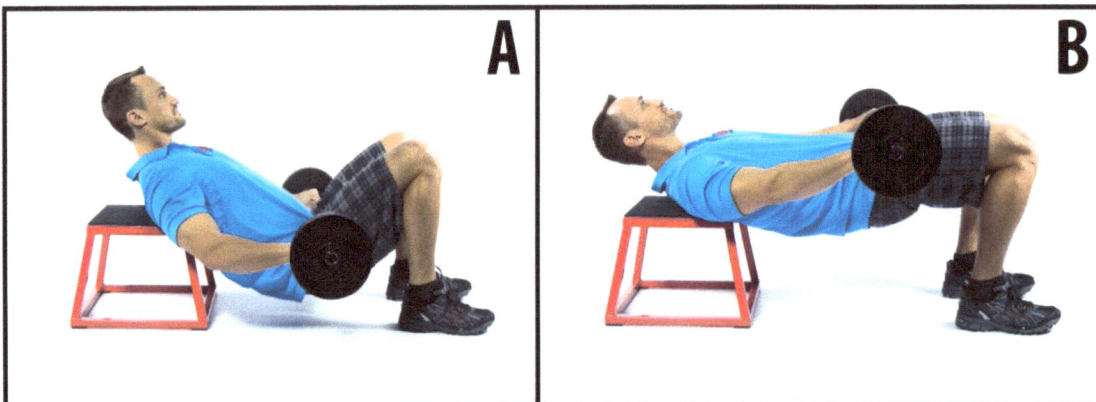

A) Start with a barbell across the upper part of the groin, just below your pelvic bone. Your feet should be pointing forward and your head in a neutral position (imagine holding an apple under your chin and you don't want to drop it!) I suggest using a towel or some sort of support as this exercise can be painful and/or leave bruising- this is normal.

B) Thrust your hips forward until your thighs are parallel to the ground. Make sure to clinch your glutes at the top. **If you want to be able to bounce a quarter off your ass aka amazing glutes, this is your go to exercise**!

Week 3: Split Routine: Chest, Shoulders, Biceps / Legs, Back, Triceps

Workout 1:	Workout2:
Bench Press	Plié Squat
Military Press	Cable Row
DB Incline Press	Leg Press
Arnold Press	Bent over Row
Bicep Curls	Tricep Extension
Accessory muscles - Bird Dogs	***Accessory muscles –*** Fire Hydrants
Walk for 20-30 minutes	Walk for 20-30 minutes at 3-3.5mph at an incline of 5-10

- 1 day of fasted cardio (30-60 minute walk/run) or AM workout
- Workout 4 days with weights + 1 day of cardio OR 1 AM workout
- 3 total sets per exercise: 12 reps (increase the weight / rest for 1 minute), 10 reps (increase the weight / rest for 1 minute), 10 reps (most difficult weight to date - move onto next exercise)
- Tempo is 1x1
- Rest 1 minute

Plié Squat

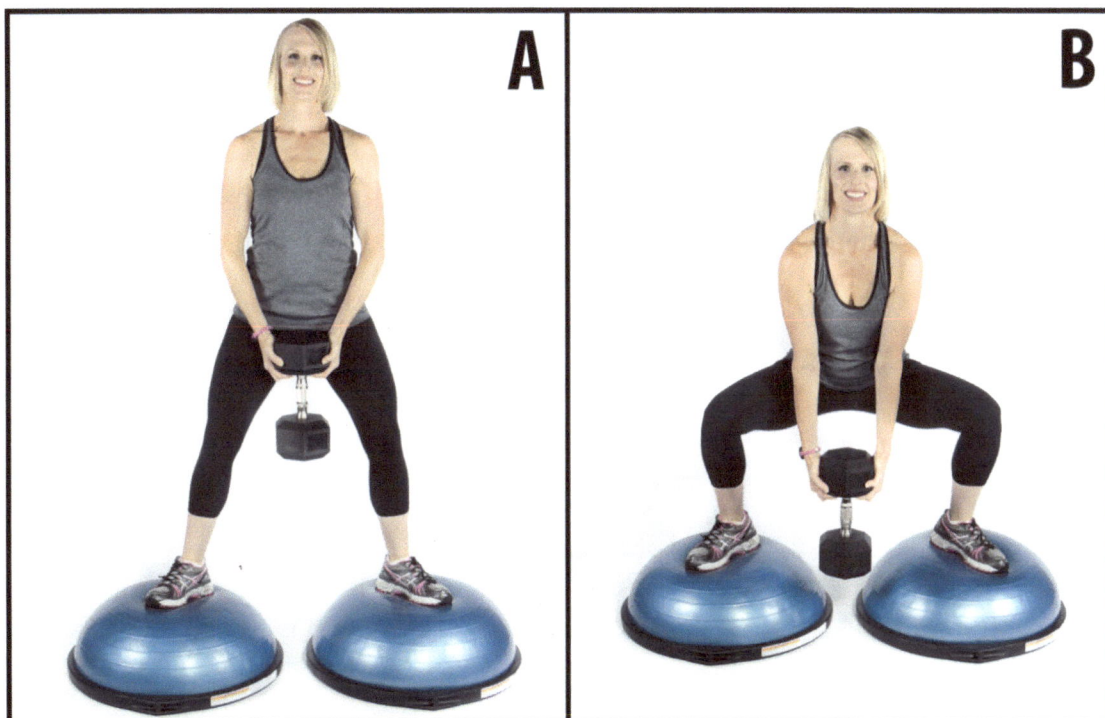

A) To begin this exercise, place your feet wider than normal and pointed at a 45 degree angle. Make sure to use a heavier than normal dumbbell- it's your legs people, they are strong! Don't pussyfoot around and grab a fucking 10lb dumbbell! My trainer here is using 40lbs and she can do this over 30 times- its super light!

B) Lower the weight until the dumbbell touches the ground. As seen in this image, she progresses the exercise by using two BOSU balls which allow her depth to increase. You could also use benches or steps to increase the potential depth.

Bird dogs:

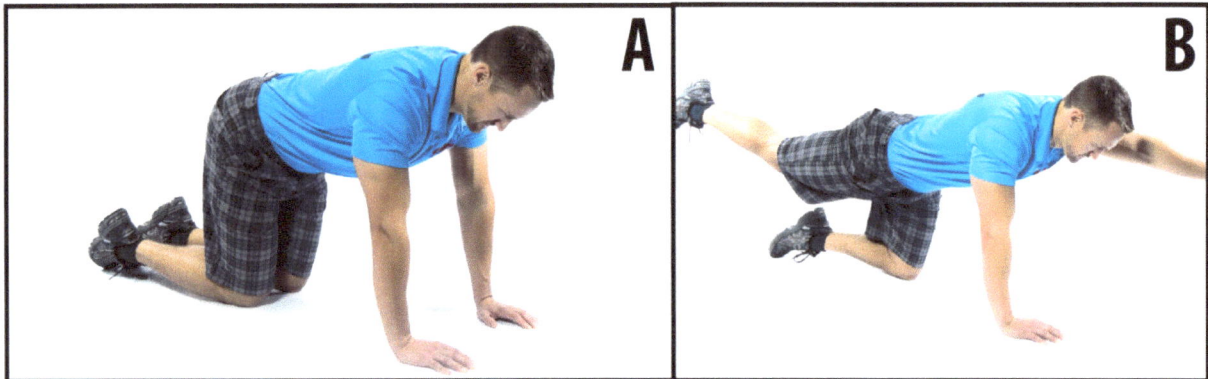

A) Begin on all fours. Your head should be in a neutral position and your core tight. Imagine a piece of string tied to your belly button and spinal column (lumbar region). To maximize core engagement, make sure you are pulling your belly button in toward your spine.

B) In a controlled manner, raise one arm and extend your opposite leg behind you. Hold for five seconds and then switch arms and legs. To make this exercise more challenging, at the end of the movement, try to touch your elbow to your opposite knee as seen in the bicycle Abs exercise.

Fire Hydrants:

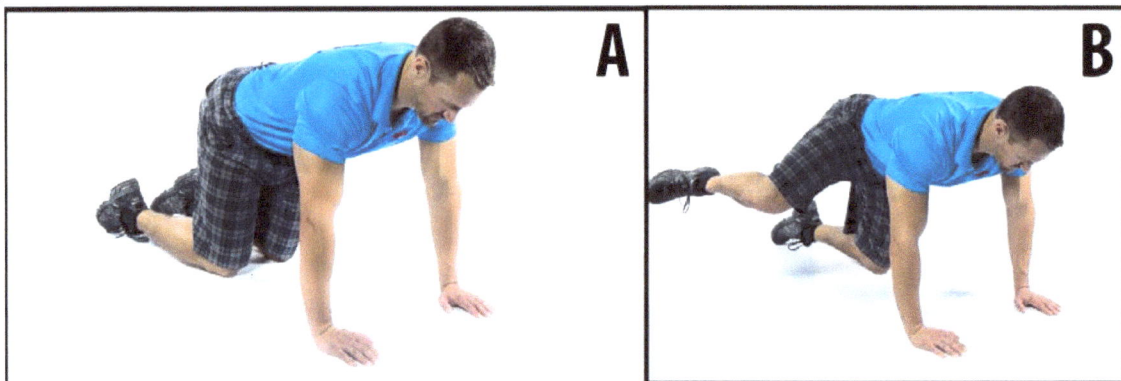

A) Begin on all fours. Your head should be in a neutral position and your core tight. Imagine a piece of string tied to your belly button and spinal column (lumbar region). To maximize core engagement, make sure you are pulling your belly button in toward your spine.

B) Raise one of your legs as if you were to take a big leak on a fire hydrant- hence the name! Keep your pelvis neutral the whole time, as you DO NOT want to rotate your hips, just your thigh aka abduction. Hold for 3 seconds.

Bent Over Row:

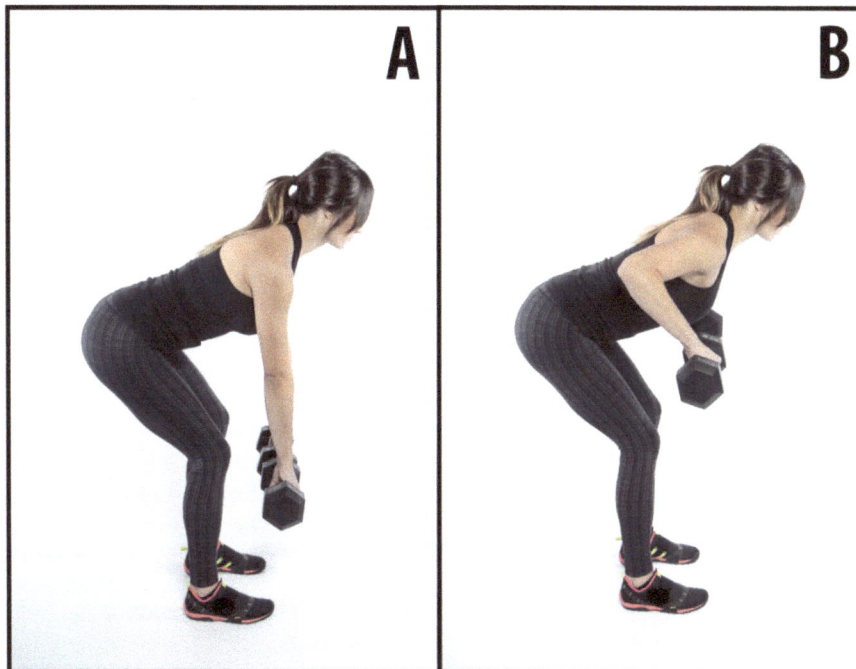

A) Begin with your body at a 45-60 degree angle. Keep your back flat and chest pressed out- think of the saying "Proud Chest". Your head should be neutral and slightly looking down. The weights should hang directly below your chest and your hands should be pronated (knuckles up).

B) Pull the weight to the sides of the chest, so the side of the dumbbell grazes the side of your chest. If you find yourself rocking and using momentum, the weight is too heavy.

AM WORKOUTS:

Perform these workouts in a circuit fashion. Exercise 1 immediately followed by exercise 2 with NO rest. I challenge you to do these before eating.

AM Workout WITHOUT weights:
30 Jumping Jacks
Max Push-ups or Negatives
Step Ups 15 per leg (chair or bed)
10 High Knees per leg
15 body weight Squats (chair or bed)
Rest 1 minute and repeat 3-5 times

AM workout WITH weights:
Lunges with shoulder press (10 per leg)
30 Jumping Jacks
15 Body weight Squats (Stability ball is better)
Max Push-ups or Negatives
Single Arm Dumbbell Row 15 per arm
10 High Knees per leg
Rest 1 minute and repeat 3-5 times

The Exercise Library:

Leg Exercises (1):
*Squat -1
Leg Press / Smith Squat- 1
Lunges- 1
Plié Squats- 1
Stability Ball Squat- 1
Romanian Deadlift (RDL) - 1
Body Weight Squats w/ weight- 1
Squat with a row- 1

Chest Exercises (2):
Bench Press-2
Incline Press-2
Dumbbell Presses-2
Chest Press Machines- 2
Weighted push-ups-2

Shoulder Exercises (3):
Military Press-3
Arnold Press-3
Face Pulls-3
Shoulder injuries/pain (4):
Upright Row (4)
Rotating T (4)

Back Exercises (5):
Lat pull-down-5
Cable row-5
Bent over row-5
Dumbbell row-5

*Squats are an awesome exercise (arguably the best). If you haven't performed this exercise before, build your base with the other exercises. IF YOU HAVE, perform squats for the next 6 weeks.

Upright Row:

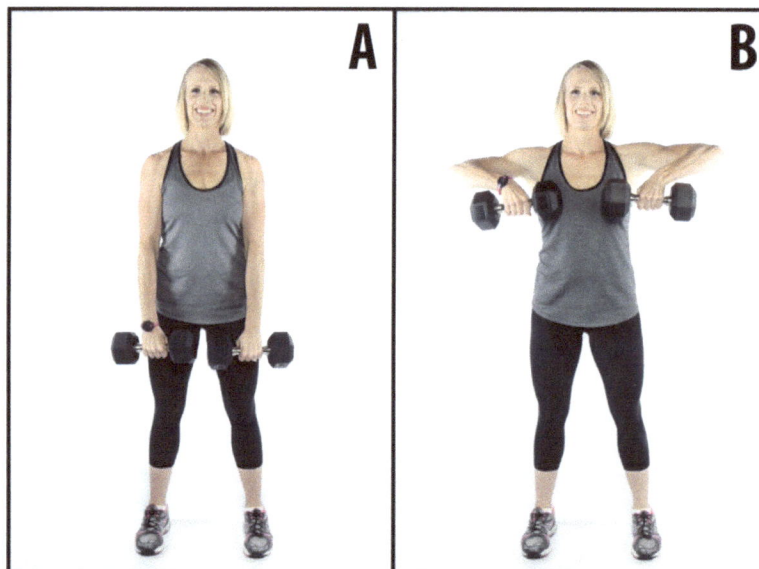

A) Begin with a big smile and either dumbbells or a barbell rest on the thighs.
B) Raise the weight to chest level. It's imperative not to raise your elbows past parallel (abduction). This will place an unwanted pressure on the rotator cuff muscle (supraspinatus). Every time you abduct the humerus past 90 degrees, you increase the likelihood of an impingement syndrome.

Lateral Raises:

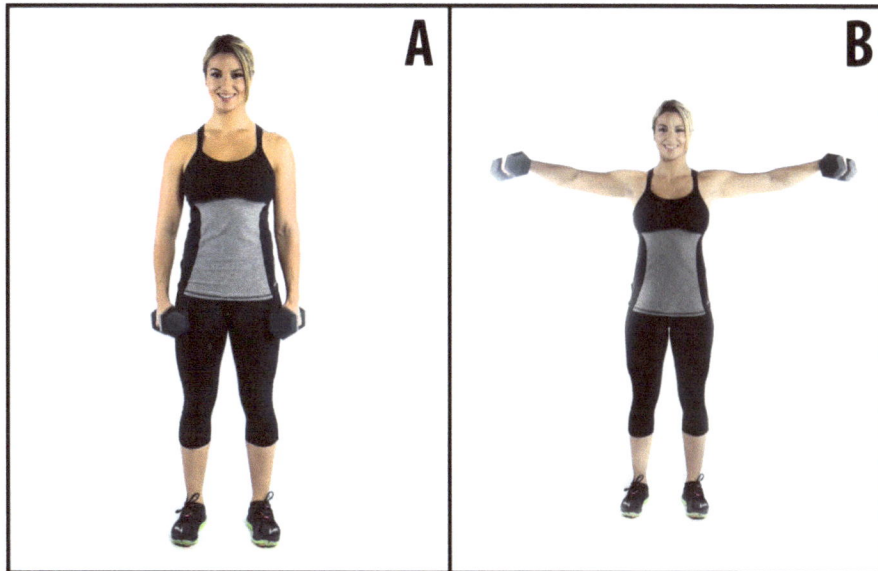

A) Begin with two dumbbells at your side.
B) In a controlled manner, raise the weights until your arm (humerus) is parallel to the ground. As seen in the previous exercise, make sure not to raise the weights above 90 degrees. This will increase the risk for an overuse syndrome of the shoulder. If you find yourself using momentum, decrease the weight.

Rotating T's:

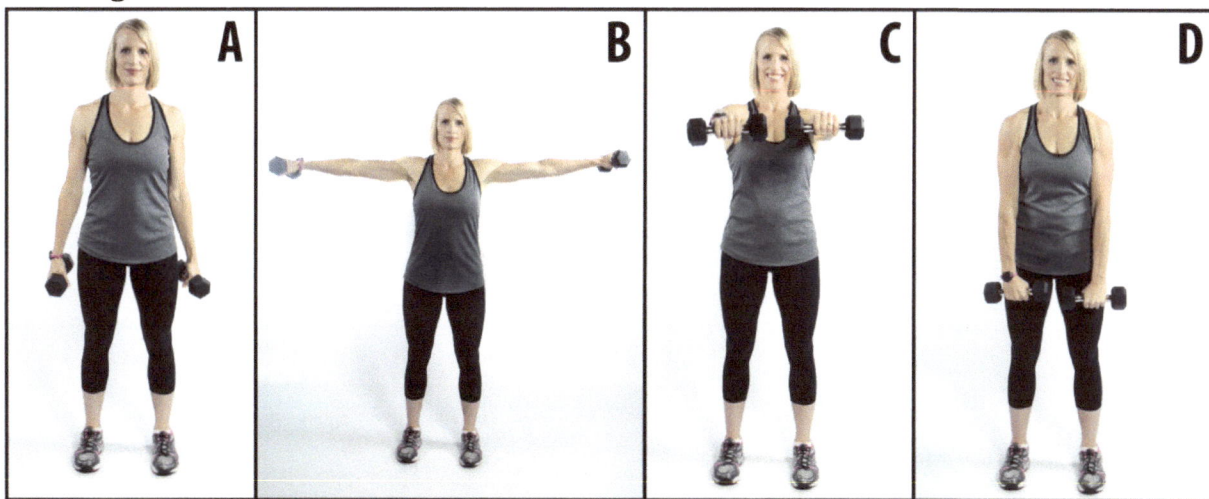

A) Begin with two weights by your side
B) Raise the weights until your arms are parallel to the ground (see lateral raise)
C) Rotate the weights forward across your body as if you were getting into a pose to be Frankenstein.
D) Lower the weights to your thighs.
   a. Repeat the steps in REVERSE order to complete ONE rep: D, C, B and finish with A.

Body weight squat with weight in front:

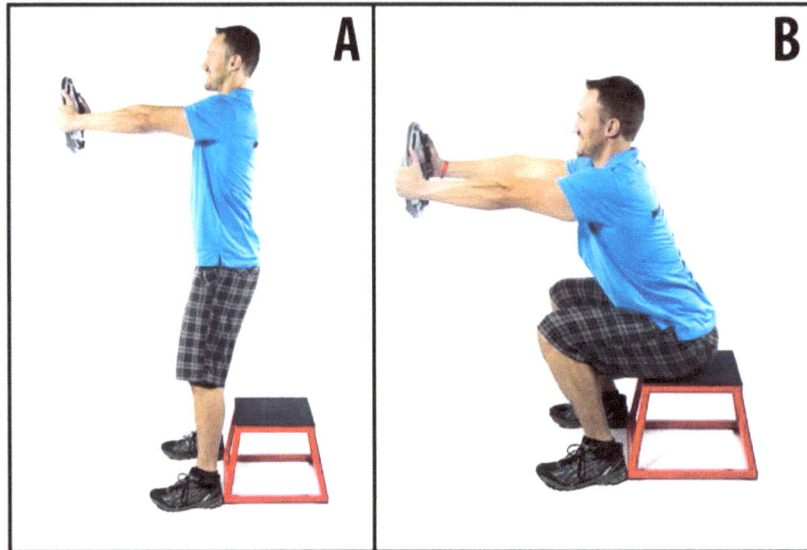

A) Begin with an 8-15lb plate or dumbbell fully extended in front of your body. The weight consciously engages your posterior muscles allowing for proper squatting technique.

B) Lower the body until your butt touches the bench. Ideally, I would like the bench to be lower than normal to maximize the engagement of the underactive glutes. I have found this exercise to be exemplary at correcting poor squatting. A common improper way to squat can be seen in the squatmorning exercise (a mixture of a good morning exercise and a squat, this isn't a good thing) where the individual flexes their core and leans over the thighs instead of maintaining an upright position as seen in the final positioning of this exercise.

Romanian Deadlift (RDL):

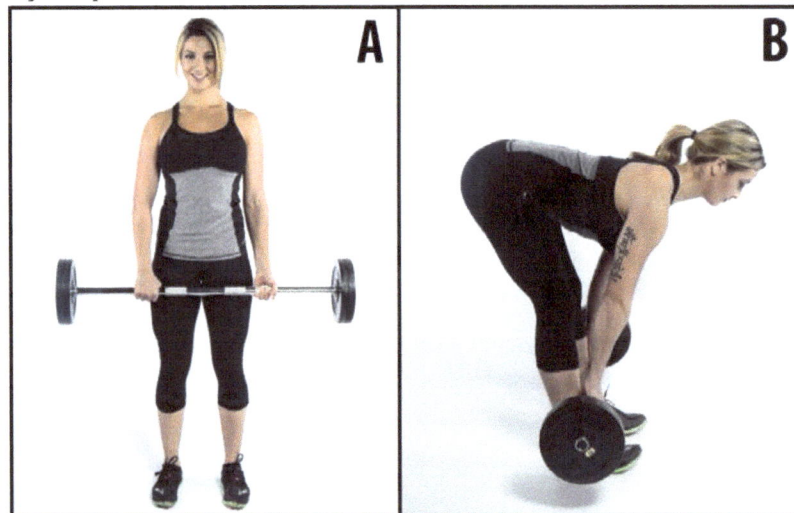

A) Begin with an alternating hand grip (one overhand and one underhand). Your feel should be in the power position (directly below your shoulders). Pinch your shoulder blades together as if you are trying to hold a card between them- Proud Shoulders!

B) The first thing you want to do it push your butt back, while keeping the bar as close to the thighs/shins as possible. Slowly lower the bar until you feel a stretch in your hamstrings. For some (usually females flexibility of the hamstrings), this stretch may not happen until the lower back goes below parallel as scene in image B. Make sure to perform this exercise near a mirror, as it is common to arch the lower back.

Lunges:

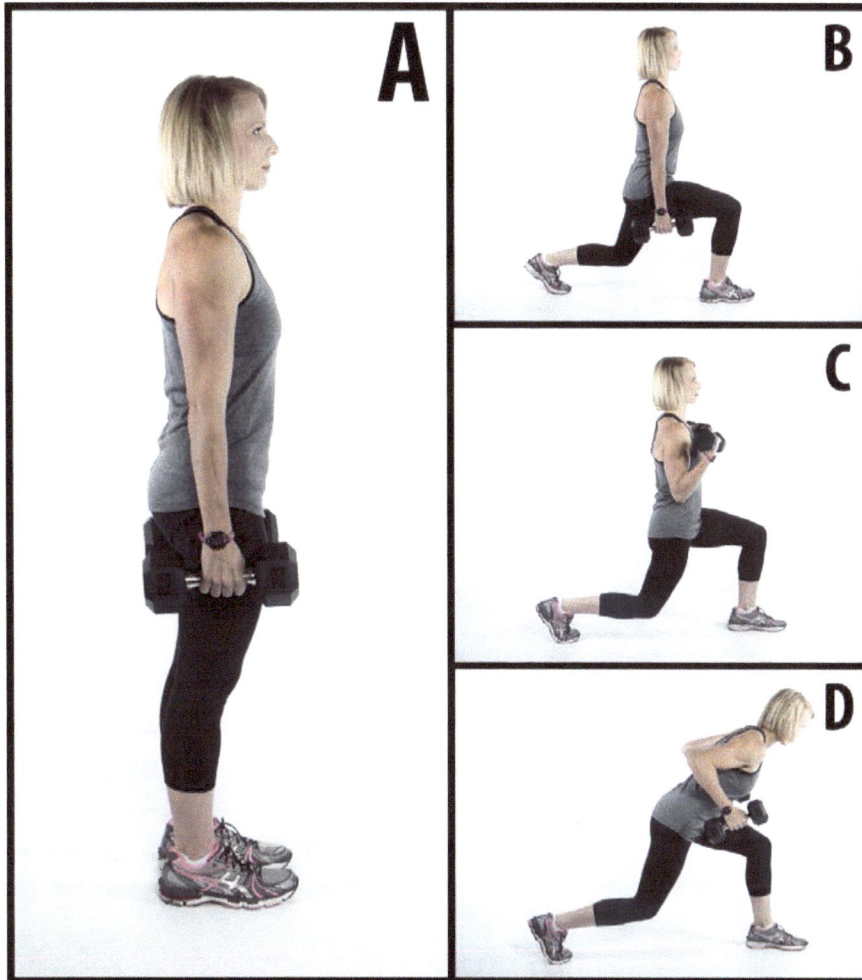

A) Begin in an upright position with your head and body neutral. You should be looking straight ahead.

B) Take a step forward. It's important not to lean forward as this is a sign that your glutes are weak and your body is innately overloading your quads to do the majority of the work. Slowly lower the trailing leg and gently touch the ground (if you are on cement, be careful as you may break your patella bone.)

    a. Either return back to your beginning position and/or walk on through to the other leg

C) Alternative options: Curl the weights on the up for a bicep curl.

    a. To maximize your glute engagement, step backwards instead of forward. By doing this (femoral extension), your glutes begin to work a lot more efficiently. Additionally, we're not use to moving backwards so we increase our proprioception aka where our body is in space.

D) At the end of the lunge, lean forward and perform a bent over row to engage your back muscles.

Push-Ups:

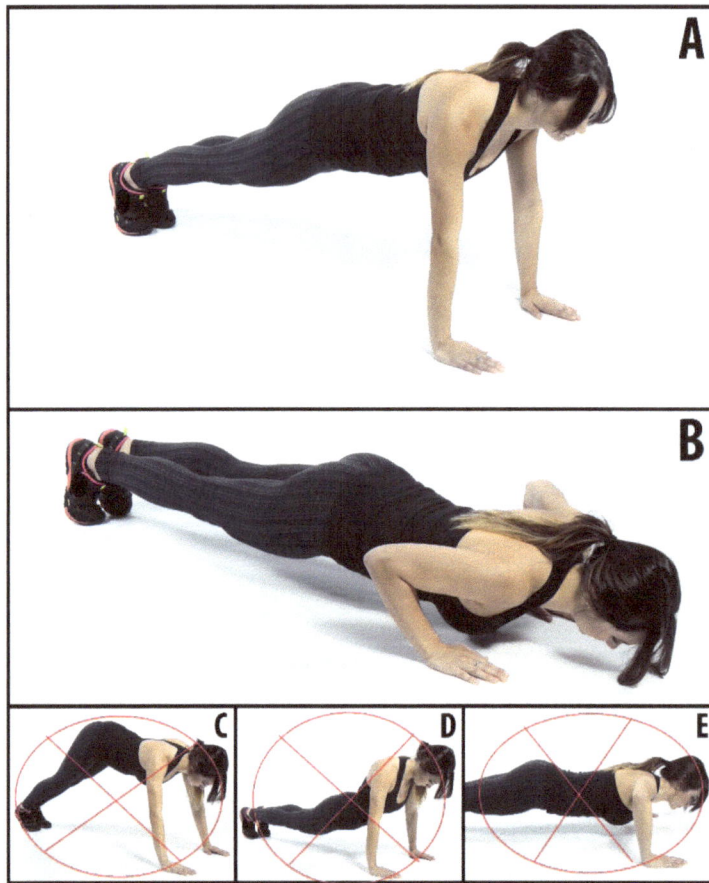

A) Begin with your hands slightly outside of shoulder width apart. Be aware, that the closer your hands are, the more emphasis will be placed on your triceps. Take a deep breath in and

B) Lower yourself to your chest touches the ground. Notice how her elbows are tucked underneath and closer to her body.

C) Avoid sticking your ass high and

D) Having your butt sink- this is a sign that you're not engaging your glutes. As I tell my clients, pretend like you're trying to wink at me with your butt cheeks- pinch those suckers hard!

E) Please don't do a 90 degree shoulder push-up. This is a trendy option as most people are not strong enough and tend to overload the shoulders. This will place a tremendous amount of pressure on your biceps tendon, potentially leading to inflammation and an overuse injury.

    a. To make this exercise easier, perform the push-up on your knees aka modified push-ups. One good push-up is better than 5 shitty ones, so don't compromise your form. If you begin to sag (D) or push your butt up (C), then go to your knees and finish them off. Remember, we all had to start somewhere!

    b. To make this exercise harder, place a weight on your middle back

Accessory muscles

Accessory muscles are any muscles other than the BIG 4 (Chest, Back, Shoulders, and Legs) Rest time = 1 minute between sets unless otherwise noted. This is where I suggest guys doing arms and/or abs while you girls focus on your thighs and arms aka your "spot reducing" areas.

- Hip Thrusters = Best Butt exercise AND low back strengthener
- Planks = Best Core exercise (hold for 15 seconds and rest for 15 seconds; repeat 4x)
- Bird Dogs = Best Balance exercise (10 per side, do not rest, just repeat the other side)
- Floor Bridges (rest for 15-30 seconds)
- Fire Hydrants (rest for 15-30 seconds)
- Shrugs (10-15 reps) - Calf raises (6-12 reps)
- Bicep Curls (10-15 reps)
- Tricep extensions (10-15 reps)
- Hip Abductors / Adductors (6-12 reps)
- ANY TYPE OF CORE EXERCISE: Side Planks/ planks, bicycle kicks.

Bicycle Kicks

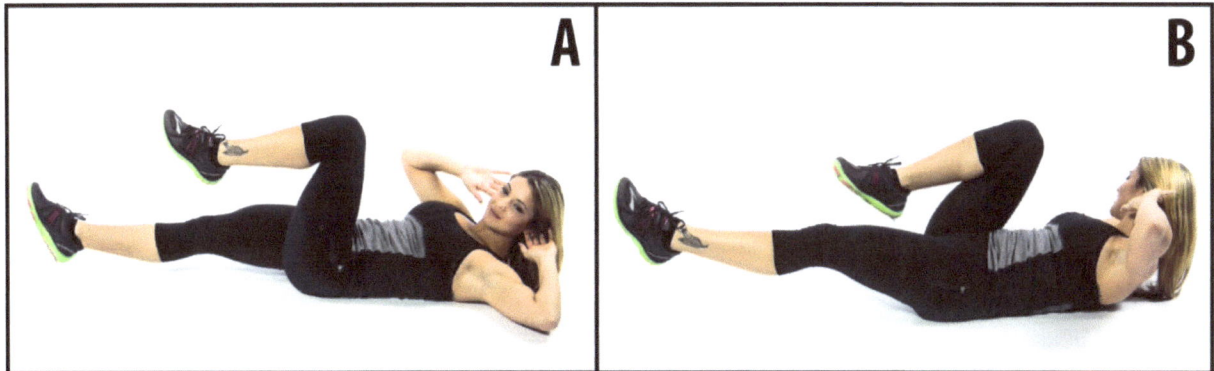

A) Begin with on your back. Cusp your ears with your hands as if you were Princess Leia. She had some radical looking bun-like-hairdo if you are unaware, so just pretend if you don't.

B) Take 3-5 seconds to rotate your right elbow and touch your left knee. Take 3-5 seconds to return to the starting position. If you are performing this exercise correctly, you should only be able to perform 2-4 reps. *Be cautious and* DON"T pull on your neck as you see in Ab infomercials!

Side Planks

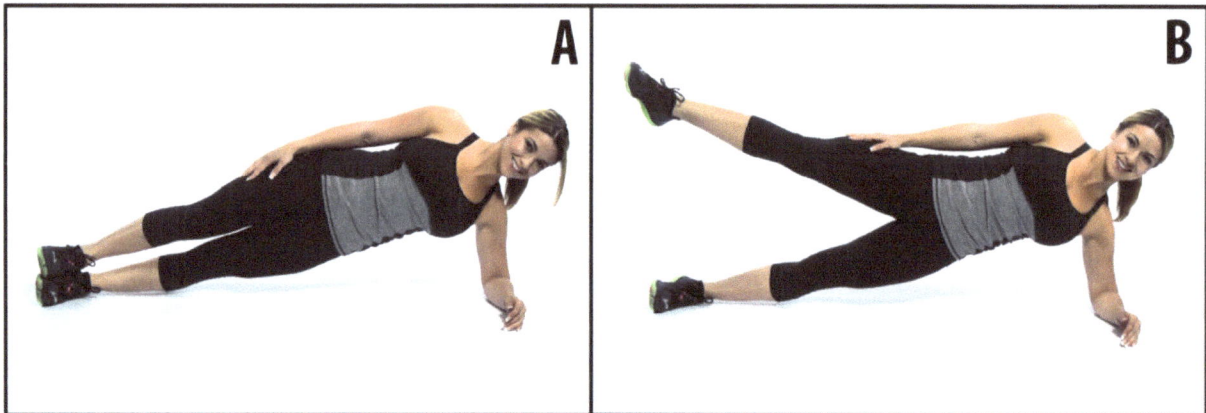

A) Begin on your side with your elbow directly under your shoulder. Keep your head in a neutral position. Clinch your butt cheeks like your trying to hold in the worlds worst smelling fart! Hold hold hold that sucker for 10-15 seconds and then switch sides.

B) To progress version A, abduct your thigh to maximize the engagement of your glutes. *Be cautious* if you have shoulder problems, I'd prefer you performing the bicycle kicks instead.

Warm up for weeks 4-6
- High Knees
- Butt Kickers
- Leg Pendulum Front / Back
- Up and Unders
- Lunges 15 per leg
- 1 set of Sumatra Push-ups
- Knee Tucks
- Planks with butt kick / abduction (10 per leg)

Week 4: Split Routine: Legs, Chest, Shoulders, Biceps / Legs, Back, Triceps

Workout 1	Workout2
Hip Thrusts	Squat (step up)
Bench Press	Cable Row
Military Press	Lunges (reverse) / (leg press)
DB Incline Press	Bent over row
Arnold Press	Tricep Extension
Accessory muscles - Bird Dogs	*Accessory muscles-* Planks
Walk OR HIIT	Walk for 20-30 minutes at 3-3.5mph @ incline of 8-12

- 1 day of fasted cardio (30-60 minute walk/run) or AM workout AND 1 day of HIIT – High Intense Interval Training: 10 seconds of sprinting rest for 1 minute. Repeat 6-8 times. May be done fasted in the morning or after workout. Make sure to perform WARM UP before.
- Workout 4 days with weights, 2 days of cardio
- Perform 4 sets increasing the weights each set: 15 reps, 12 reps, 10 reps, 10 reps (DROP SET). During set #4, you will aim for performing 20 TOTAL reps. Use the same weight you used for set 3 and perform maximal reps. After fatigue, you will immediately lower the weight to an amount you can perform consecutively for the remaining reps. It is likely you will fall short due to fatigue, so drop the weight again to hit that lucky number of 20 total reps for set #4.
- Tempo is 1x1
- Rest 1 minute (Rest between 60-90 for the last drop set)

Week 5: SUPER SETS: Perform each exercise set consecutively, then rest

Workout1	Workout2
Bench press	Squats
Bent over-rows	Military press
Incline DB	Lunges
DB Row	Face pulls
Bench press2	RDL (Deadlift)
Cable row2	*Accessory muscles* - Planks
Walk for 20-30	Squats2
	Military Press2
	Walk for 20-30 minutes at 3-3.5mph @ incline of 5-10

- 2 days of HIIT: 15-20 seconds of sprinting rest for 2 minutes. Repeat 6-8 times. May be done fasted in the morning or after workout.
- Workout 4 days with weights, 2 days of cardio
- Perform 5 sets increasing the weights each set: 12 reps, 10 reps, 8 reps, 6 reps, 10 reps - Aim for 20 total reps for the exercise group. I.E. Lat Pull-Downs 6 reps, Bent over rows 14 reps, then rest.
- For the exercises labeled 2: Perform one large drop set for 30 reps at the end. Find a weight you can perform 8-10 reps then immediately lower the weight and aim for 8-12 reps then lower again and then finish off the remainder of the reps.
- Tempo is 1x1 (1 second down and 1 second up)
- Rest 60-90 seconds

Week 6: COMPOUND SETS: Perform each exercise set consecutively, then rest

Workout1	Workout2
Bench press	Squats
Push-ups	Lunges
Lat pull-downs	Military press
Cable row	Face pulls
Bench press2	RDL (Deadlift)
Lat pull-downs2	*Accessory muscles- Bird dogs*
Accessory muscles –Planks	Lunges with weights2
Walk for 20-30 minutes OR HIIT	Military press2
	Walk 20-30 minutes at 3-3.5mph + incline of 5-10

- Perform 5 sets increasing the weights each set: 12 reps, 10 reps, 8 reps, 6 reps, 10 reps. For the second exercise, aim for 8-12 reps or go until fatigue i.e. push-ups.
- For the exercises labeled 2: Perform TWO large drop set for 30 reps. Find a weight you can perform 8-10 reps, same for set 2 and then finish off the remainder of the reps. Rest for 1-2 minutes and perform one more set.
- Tempo is 1x1
- Rest 1-2 minutes (Rest 2 minutes between the drop sets)

Week 7: *Detrain OR choose your favorite workout from previous 6 weeks and perform 4-6 times*

Week 8 / 9:
Workout 1: Chest and Back
Bench Press 4 sets of 8 rest 1 min
Lat pull down 4 sets of 8 rest 1 min
Incline Dumbbell Press 4 sets of 10 rest 30 seconds
Cable row 4 sets of 10 rest 30 seconds
3 sets of Max push-ups
3 sets of assisted pull-up machine or Band pull-ups 10-15 reps
Side Planks
Walk for 20-30 minutes

Workout 2: Legs and arms
Jump Squats (if your knees permit) 10 max jumps, followed immediately by 1 minute of (choose one) jumping jacks/jump rope/step ups. After 1 min. of cardio, rest 1 minute and repeat x 4 sets
Squats 4 sets of 8 rest one minute
Dumbbell Bicep curls 3 sets of 10; tricep push-downs 3 sets of 10 (super set, no rest between bi / tri) rest 1 min after
Lunges 4 sets of 10 per leg rest one minute
Bicep curl (bar or machine) 3 sets of 10; tricep push-down 3 sets of 10 (super set, no rest between bi / tri) rest 1 min after
RDL 4 sets of 10 rest one minute
ABS (Choose any ab exercise)
Walk for 20-30 minutes

Jump Squats:

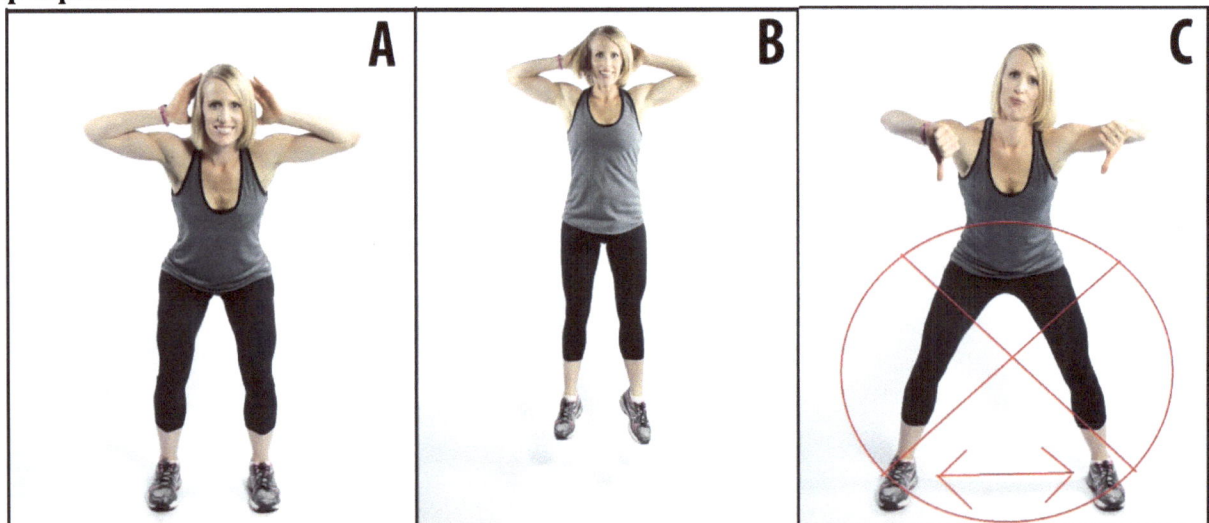

A) Begin with your hands behind your head and your legs directly under your shoulders in the power position. Power and strength are different. To maximize vertical height, your legs should be closer in (A) and not further out (C). Squat down to a 1/4th of a squat and recoil by

B) Jumping up as high as you can! Try not to lean forward. If you notice that your knees bend in (knee valgus), then we need to strengthen your glutes via hip thrusters, lunges and squats.

Workout 3: Shoulders
Military Press (seated or machine) 4 sets of 8 rest one minute
Arnold Press 4 sets of 10 rest one minute (weight should be lighter than military)
Lateral Raises (side shoulder raise with dumbbell) 4 sets of 12 rest one minute
Upright rows 4 sets of 10 rest one minute
Lower Back extensions 3 sets of 15 rest one minute
Walk for 20-30 minutes

Workout 4: Full body
Max jumps 10 (if knees permit) Lunges 10 per leg rest one minute x four sets
Max Push-ups; Bent over rows 4 sets of 10 (super set, no rest between push and row) rest one minute
Lat Pull-downs 4 sets of 10 rest one minute
Standing military press with dumbbells; lateral raises (super set) 4 sets of 10 each
1 minute of (choose one) jumping jacks/jump rope/step ups on a bench followed by 15 second plank (remember to clinch your glutes) x five sets
Day 5 & 6 optional: Repeat one of your favorite workouts

Week 10:

Day 1: Cardio Day

Dynamic Warm Up (as seen in the first 1-3 weeks) 5 minutes
Max push-ups (modified aka girly push-ups or regular push-ups. Perform as many as you can)
Cardio of your choice (I suggest walking at an incline, biking, elliptical or running) - 10 minutes
Max Push-ups (get off treadmill and perform push-ups)
High Intense Interval Training 10-15 seconds of maximal effort, followed by 1-2 minutes of rest for 2-3 sets - 8-10 minutes
Max Push-ups (get off treadmill and perform push-ups)
High Intense Interval Training 10-15 seconds of maximal effort, followed by 1-2 minutes of rest for 2-3 sets - 8-10 minutes
Max Push-ups (get off treadmill and perform push-ups)
Cardio of your choice (I suggest walking at an incline, biking, elliptical or running) - 10 minutes
Max Push-ups (get off treadmill and perform push-ups)

Total: 5 max push-up sets. 2 Interval sets for a total of 16-20 minutes (6 total sets), 2 cardio sessions of walking, jogging, biking etc for a total of 20 minutes. REST WHEN NEEDED

Day 2: Full Body
Legs: Squats / Lunges / Leg Press / Plie Squats (Choose 1) 5 sets. First set 15 reps, add weight rest 30 seconds, 12 reps, add weight rest 30 seconds, 10 reps, add weight rest 1 minute, 8 reps, add weight rest one minute, end with 6 reps. If you can do more than 6 reps, weight is TOO LIGHT!!!
Chest: Bench Press / Incline Dumbbells / Chest Press Machine (Choose 1). Same as above
Back: Cable Row / Lat Pulldown / T Bar Row / Bent over row (Choose 1).Same as above
Shoulders: Military Press / Upright Row / Arnold Press / Shoulder Press Machine (Choose 1).
Biceps & Triceps: Perform 1 bicep exercise and immediately follow it with a tricep exercise.
Core circuit (do this circuit 3-5 times): 15 seconds of jumping jacks. Abs crunches 10 reps. 15 seconds of jumping jacks. Weighted side bends (10 per side - grab dumbbells and bend at the side). 15 seconds of jumping jacks. Planks (remember to clinch your BUTT for 15 seconds.) 15 seconds of jumping jacks.

Day 3: Burpee Cardio

Dynamic Warm up - 5 minutes
Cardio of your choice (I suggest walking) 3 minutes
5 burpees (get off of cardio equipment)
Cardio of your choice (I suggest walking) 3 minutes
5 burpees (get off of cardio equipment)

Do 10 sets for a total of 50 burpees and 30 minutes of walking

After, I highly suggest performing lunges, push-ups and assisted pull-up machine for 3-5 sets of 10 reps

Day 4: Full Body

Legs: Suitcase Squats / Lunges / Leg Press / Plie Squats (Choose 1) 5 sets. First set 15 reps, add weight rest 30 seconds, 12 reps, add weight rest 30 seconds, 10 reps, add weight rest 1 minute, 8 reps, add weight rest one minute, end with 6 reps. If you can do more than 6 reps, weight is TOO LIGHT!!!
Chest: Bench Press / Incline Dumbbells / Chest Press Machine (Choose 1). Same as above
Back: Cable Row / Lat Pulldown / T Bar Row / Bent over row (Choose 1).Same as above
Shoulders: Military Press / Upright Row / Arnold Press / Shoulder Press Machine (Choose 1).
Biceps & Triceps: Perform 1 bicep exercise and immediately follow it with a tricep exercise.
Core circuit (do this circuit 3-5 times): 15 seconds of jumping jacks. Abs crunches 10 reps. 15 seconds of jumping jacks. Weighted side bends (10 per side - grab dumbbells and bend at the side). 15 seconds of jumping jacks. Planks (remember to clinch your BUTT for 15 seconds.) 15 seconds of jumping jacks.
Day 5 & 6 optional: Repeat favorite workout

Suitcase Squats (C):

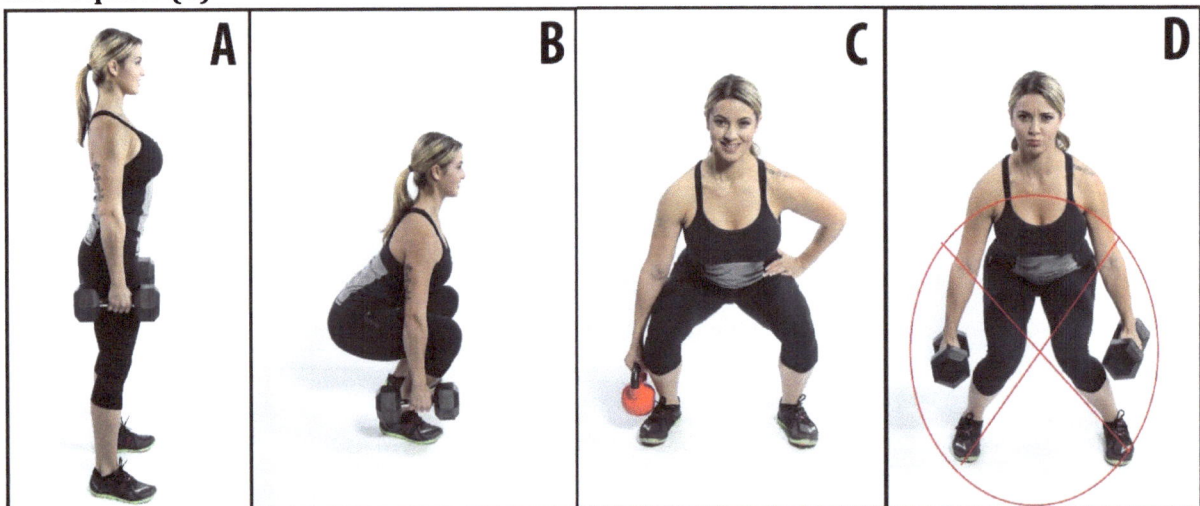

A) Regular dumbbell squat: Begin with the dumbbell's at your side. Have your toes slightly pointed out (10-15 degrees). This isn't very much; it's about the size of a big toe. Not Bigfoots big toe, just a regular one, so don't overemphasize.

B) Lower the weights until your thighs are at least parallel to the ground and/or your tail end begins to tuck under. See how Lindsey's back is straight and not arched? That's a perfect squat.

C) This is a suitcase squat. How do you carry a suitcase to the airport? Bingo! This exercise is the same as the squat; instead, you only use one dumbbell or Kettlebells. By doing so, you engage your core a lot more.

D) If your knees buckle, imagine your feet in cement and try pulling your knees apart. By doing so, you initiate external rotation which engages the glutes and deep six rotators. This will stabilize the hip and correct your poor squatting. D is also a sign that your glutes are weak, so revert back to floor bridges, lunges, hip thrusters and remember to clinch your ass whenever you can!

Week 11 workout
You'll be performing 4 sets while doing the following style for the reps: warm up for 15 reps. Add weight that you can only perform enough reps for 10 reps; add enough weight where you can only do 8 reps. Last set, add enough weight where you can only do 6 reps (should be the heaviest to date with proper form.) When you complete the 6th rep, drop the weight to an amount that you can perform 10 additional reps (drop set.) Rest between sets 30-60 seconds. You'll see this is a combo of the previous 3 weeks...

Workout 1: Chest and Back
Bench Press
Lat pull down
Incline Dumbbell Press or incline machine
Bent over barbell row (Stand at a 45 degree angle and pull bar to lower part of chest.)
After weights... CARDIO... for 30 minutes
Dynamic Warm Up (as seen in the first 1-3 weeks) 5 minutes
Cardio of your choice (I suggest walking at an incline, biking, elliptical or running) – 5 minutes
Max Push-ups (get off treadmill and perform push-ups)
High Intense Interval Training 10-15 seconds of maximal effort, followed by 1-2 minutes of rest for 2-3 sets - 8-10 minutes
Max Push-ups (get off treadmill and perform push-ups)
High Intense Interval Training 10-15 seconds of maximal effort, followed by 1-2 minutes of rest for 2-3 sets - 8-10 minutes
Max Push-ups (get off treadmill and perform push-ups)
Cardio of your choice (I suggest walking at an incline, biking, elliptical or running) – 5 minutes
Max Push-ups (get off treadmill and perform push-ups)

Workout 2: Shoulders
Military Press (seated or machine)
Arnold Press 4 sets of 10 rest one minute
Lateral Raises (side shoulder raise with dumbbell)
Upright rows 4 sets of 10 rest one minute
Lower Back extensions 3 sets of 15 rest one minute
Cardio for 30 minutes....

Burpee Cardio
Dynamic Warm up - 5 minutes
Cardio of your choice (I suggest walking) 3 minutes
5 burpees (get off of cardio equipment)
Cardio of your choice (I suggest walking) 3 minutes
5 burpees (get off of cardio equipment)
Do 10 sets for a total of 50 burpees and 30 minutes of walking

Workout 3: Legs and Arms
Jump Squats (if your knees permit) 10 max jumps, followed immediately by 1 minute of (choose one) jumping jacks/jump rope/step ups. After 1 min. of cardio, rest 1 minute and repeat x 4 sets
Squats
Dumbbell Bicep curls 3 sets of 10; tricep push-downs 3 sets of 10 (super set, no rest between bi / tri) rest 1 min after
Lunges
Bicep curl (bar or machine) 3 sets of 10; tricep push-down 3 sets of 10 (super set, no rest between bi / tri) rest 1 min after
RDL 4 sets of 10 rest one minute
ABS (Choose any ab exercise)
Walk for 20-30 minutes OR Choose Favorite Cardio Day

Workout 4:
Legs: Squats / Lunges / Leg Press / Plie Squats (Choose 1)
Chest: Bench Press / Incline Dumbbells / Chest Press Machine (Choose 1)
Back: Cable Row / Lat Pulldown / T Bar Row / Bent over row (Choose 1)
Shoulders: Military Press / Upright Row / Arnold Press / Shoulder Press Machine
Biceps & Triceps: Perform 1 bicep exercise and immediately follow it with a tricep exercise.
Core circuit (do this circuit 3-5 times): 15 seconds of jumping jacks. Abs crunches 10 reps. 15 seconds of jumping jacks. Weighted side bends (10 per side - grab dumbbells and bend at the side). 15 seconds of jumping jacks. Planks (remember to clinch your BUTT for 15 seconds.) 15 seconds of jumping jacks.
Walk for 30 minutes OR choose favorite CARDIO DAY

Workouts 5&6 optional: Repeat favorite workout

Week 12 workout: Repeat x2 (aim for 6 days)
Day 1:
Squats 5 sets of 6-8 reps
single leg explosive (8 per leg)

Bench Press 6-8 reps
ball pushes chest

RDL 6-8
Max jumps 5

Incline dumbbell
Push-ups
20 min walk

Single Leg Explosive:

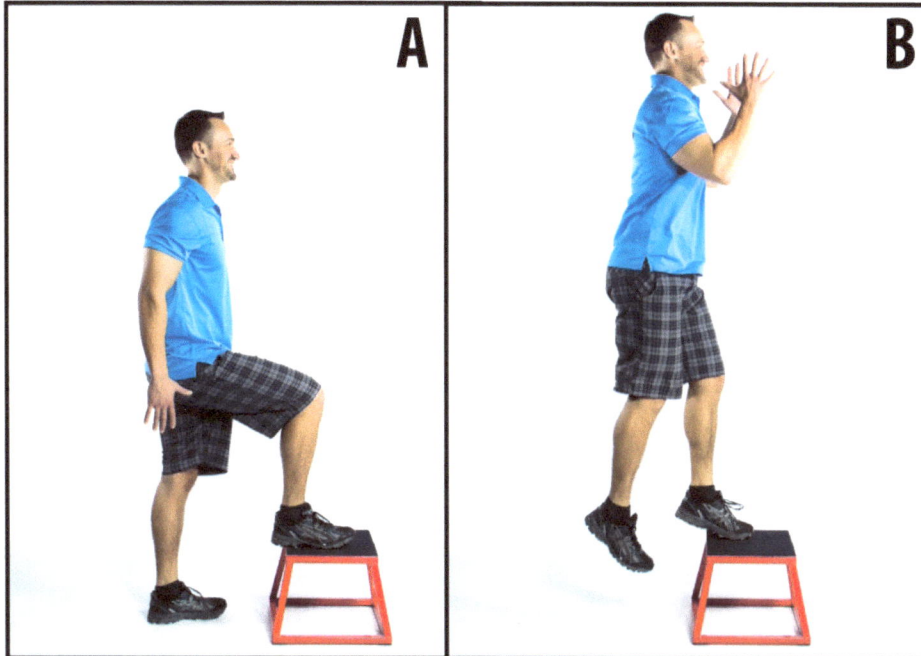

A) Begin with one leg on a plyo box / bench or chair.

B) Explosively swing your hands forward and jump straight up into the air. While in the air, you are going to switch legs and land on the opposite leg and repeat the exercise. Your arms contribute roughly 20% of total force production, so make sure to swing them forward to maximize the height.

    a. This exercise is definitely more advanced. Make sure to watch the videos on my website to make sure you are doing them correctly.

Med Ball Push:

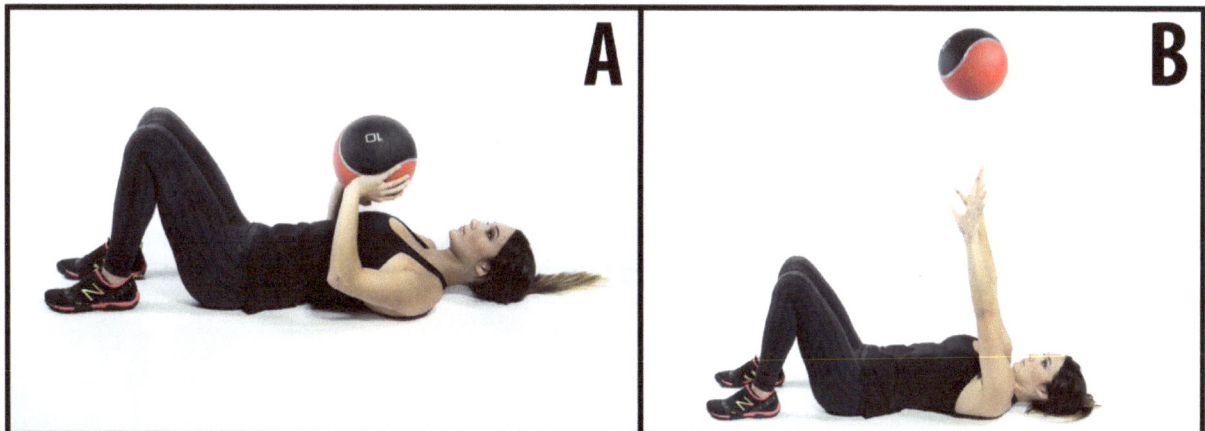

A) Begin on your back with a medicine ball that weighs between 5-15lbs resting on your chest.

B) As hard as you can, push the ball into the air. I like to have my clients and students perform this exercise in a room with 20+ foot ceilings. I encourage them to try and hit the ceiling to encourage maximal power production.

    a. This exercise is fun, but you might want to have a spotter catch the ball. Be careful of that pretty face, don't let the ball smash it on its way down!

Day 2:
Cable row
Ball slam

Military press
Ball push (Same as med ball chest push, but you push the ball overhead in a standing postion)

Lat pull down
Bent over row

Rotation T
Upright row

Precore HIIT 6 sets of 10-15 seconds. Rest 60-90 seconds between sets

Ball Slam:

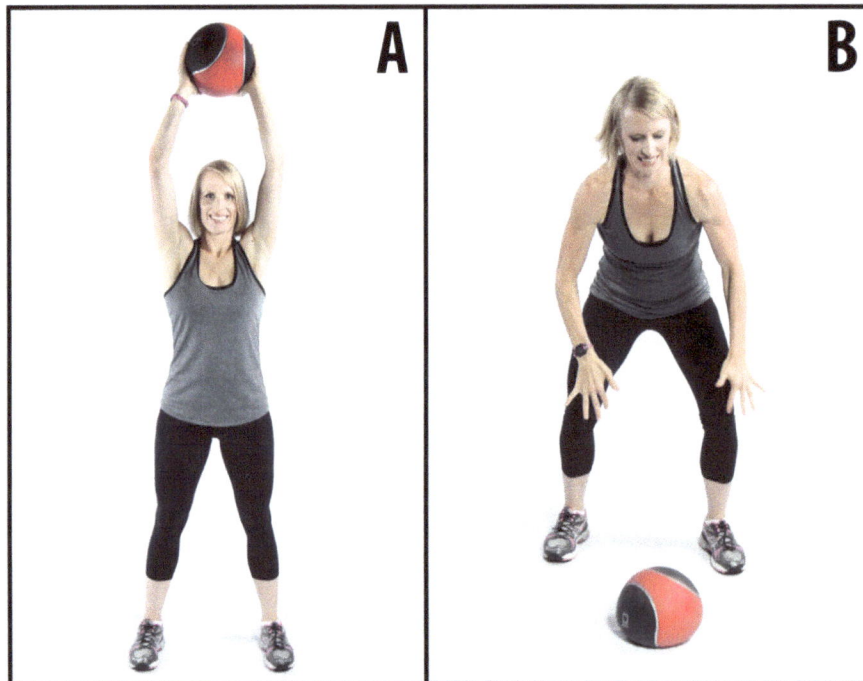

A) Begin with a medicine ball above your head. *Be cautious* because there are many medicine balls. Some bounce and others do not. Please don't hit yourself in the fucking face and blame The VTD for it, that's your fault for being a dumbass!
B) Slam the ball into the ground as hard as you possibly can.
   a. I suggest using a ball that weighs between 5-12lbs. FYI, look how freaking tough Leah is, she pretty much smashed the ball into oblivion!

DAY3: Circuit days repeat 2-3times
Circuits:
Lunges
Burpees
Push-ups
Abs

Step ups w curl
bent over rows triceps
Jumping jacks
Planks

Squat w/ press
Ball tap
Hip thrusts
Bicycle abs

Ball Tap:

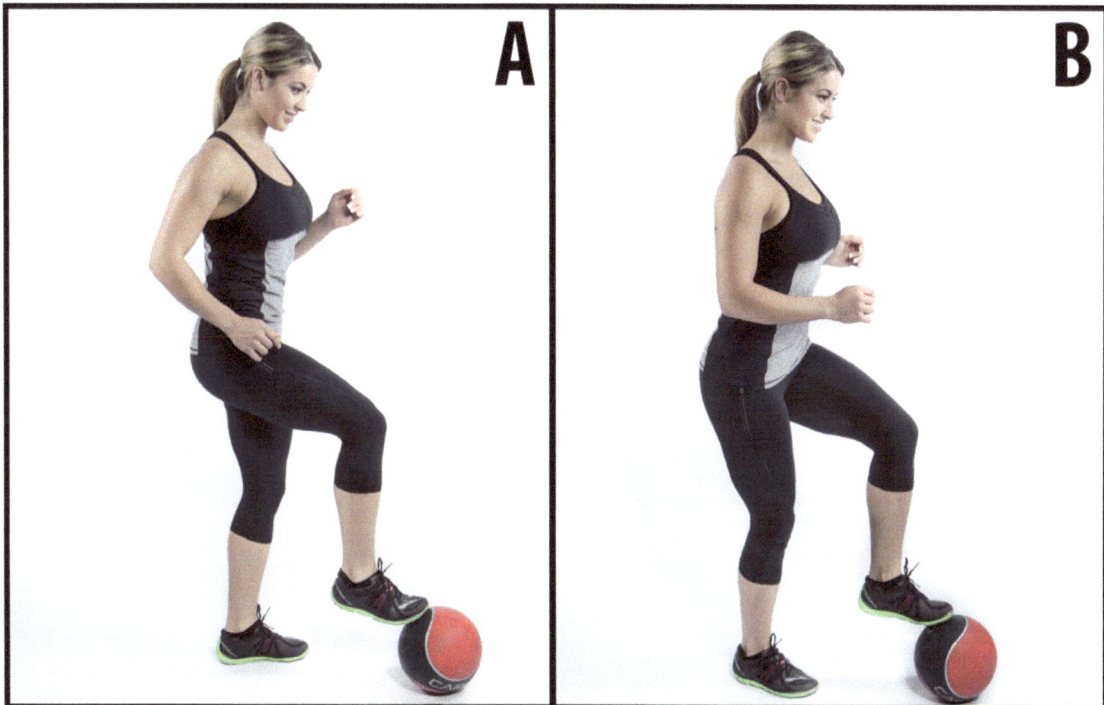

A) A med ball / cone / dumbbell will suffice for this cardio exercise. Tap the ball as quickly as you can and

B) Switch to the other foot. I prefer a med ball because the chances of it rolling increase. This is beneficial because the brain enjoys tracking down objects by releasing the protein BDNF. Remember this sucker increases neuroplasticity.

Breakdown and Expectations

<u>What to expect weeks 1-6</u>:

When you head into basic training, you are preparing for the worst; do the same here. I am not going to sugar coat it, the first 4-6 weeks will suck. If it helps, just imagine jumping into a freezing lake ass naked; yeah, I know it doesn't sound appealing. After a few minutes, you will acclimate and be able to stomach the rest. If you stick it out, your choices and behaviors will change for the better.

Don't expect immediate results. You will not morph into the unreal people you see on TV. I swear the people you see on TV are fake; where the fuck are they in our everyday lives? There must be some fictitious planet out there streaming video to our TVs because I never ever see crazy-in-shape people walking the streets, except my girlfriend- (brownie points!)

It is important to note that all the benefits that I stated about exercise are true, but it takes time to reveal them. Understand that you're not alone. There will be people who quit and give up; it's expected. They usually stop within the first couple of weeks because they aren't looking better, or their body feels worse. Constant soreness and a decline in energy may be a deterrent. It takes some time for your body to adapt to a new stimulus. Half of the battle is showing up. Stick through this for 30 days, and the likelihood for your success will dramatically increase. At the end of 30 days, you will be able to look back and will definitely notice a difference.

I want the first few weeks to be realistic, so we will be using lighter weights: 12-20 reps. I want to encourage activity, so we will be aiming for three to four resistance training sessions per week. If you're a go-getter, do more; the more the merrier! Remember, the body needs at least one day of rest. I suggest sitting down and using the calendar to mark the days you are going to workout. A detailed calendar will mitigate the chances of quitting. Spend an hour at the office filling it out, and your boss will think you're hard at work. This is your "me" time, and don't let anyone mess with it! Remember when you were a little kid and for Christmas you got a brand-new teddy bear? What did you do to that teddy bear? You held him, you loved him, and most importantly, you wouldn't let anyone fuck with teddy! If anyone tries to compromise your workouts, don't get flustered! Just come back to your calendar and adjust it.

We are using light weights to strengthen ligaments and tendons (connective tissue). After these first few weeks, the body will want more, and weeks 3-6 allow for this. The volume will be amplified during weeks 4-6 because your body is now ready for the extra load. Progressing too fast sets the body up for an injury.

One to two pounds of fat loss or 1% of bodyweight loss a week is wack-a-doodle-doo amazing! When we factor in a little muscle growth, a net scale loss of three to six pounds is par for the course for part one. Anything additional is wack-a-doodle-doo amazing! When was the last time you said that word twice in one day? Well, get ready for a third! You're wack-a-doodle-doo fucking amazing if you lose three to six pounds in the first six weeks! How many plans suggest this? Not many, and that's what some many people fail from: unrealistic results!

If your SPI portion of the S.P.I.N.E score completely blows, your body may be giving you the middle finger by signaling itself to hold onto fat. When your stress levels are high, cortisol won't let your body lose fat. Fat is the highest yielding fuel for the body, so it'll store it instead of burning it. To make matters worse, you'll probably burn muscle instead. I know this sounds horrible, because it is. It will continue to happen until SPI portion is properly addressed, primarily better sleep and less stress. If this is you, don't expect any scale loss. The most important determinant if you're this type person is not giving up. Continue to eat well, drink water, and exercise minimally. Yes, minimally. Maybe three days of weights and limit the cardio sessions to 30 minutes. Exercise is stress, so I want to avoid overtraining. Addressing these issues will be paramount for your fat loss success. Seeking therapy and/or a doctor who specializes in hormonal imbalance or adrenal fatigue may be your best bet. It's like you're stuck in mud. Working out harder will only dig yourself deeper in the hole and this book can only do so much to help get you out. After a while, a specialist may be needed. Once the issues are addressed, hop back on the VTD plan, and you'll be able to cruise along to your fat loss goals!

Weeks 1-3 to maximize fat loss: Aim for cardio or the AM workouts three times a week outside of the 3-4 resistance workouts. Wake up in the morning and do fasted cardio for 30-60 minutes or find 30-60 minutes during lunch or after dinner.

Weeks 4-6 to maximize fat loss: Aim for 2 days of HIIT training, and after the HIIT training walk for 20-30 minutes for 60 total minutes. (HIIT should take 20-30 / walk after 20-30 = 60 minutes)

Weeks 7-12:
Week seven may throw some of you guys off. A detraining week, WTF? Even though you may be rocking toward your fat loss goals, think of it as six steps forward and then pausing to gather yourself, and then repeat. This is a built-in mechanism I added to prevent any injuries. I call week seven the injury buster. If you are feeling awesome, I encourage you to choose one of the workouts from the previous six weeks and repeat: no harm, no foul. One common mistake I see with beginners is the urge to give 110%, the all-or-nothing mentality. This mentality is exactly what I love to see, but proper periodization has built in days and weeks for rest. Rest is a lot like sleep. If you don't implement into your workout plan, you're going to burn out!

After this week, we advance into the rest of the workout schedule with higher intensity workouts. This is when we start having fun! Cardio, burpees, sprints, and awesome split routines. Your clothes will be fitting better, and the compliments will be running high. The optimal goal is to reduce body fat while reconditioning the body to handle a higher workload in a safely and properly progressed manner.

Weeks 8-9 to maximize fat loss: Aim for two days of HIIT training and one day of fasted cardio or AM workouts outside of the workout schedule.

Weeks 10-12 to maximize fat loss: Aim for three days of fasted cardio or AM workouts outside of the workout schedule.

Anything outside of this workout schedule can be implemented to complement this system. If you want to take a spin class, Zumba, or any other sort of aerobics class instead of the fasted cardio - have at it! Be that good friend, and encourage your circle of friends to start walking with you in the morning. Holding each other accountable will increase your chances of fat loss. I highly suggest classes like Yoga, Pilates, and tai chi, but they will not replace any workouts or cardio; they will just help fix your S.P.I.N.E.™.

What's Next After I Finish the VTD Workouts?
First off, I want to congratulate you on the hard ass work you put in. Second, go show off your new bod by buying some clothes and treating yourself to something really nice!

What's next? Back to the old habits and turning into Pigzilla? No. We need to continue this healthy lifestyle that you have adopted. If you still have more fat to lose, go back through the workouts 4-12 and pick your favorite ones. Implement week 7 every 6-8 weeks for a week of detraining, which will allow your body to rest. Many of my students and clients discover that after this week off, they come back healthier, stronger, and re-energized

How to fix your S.P.I.N.E.™:

Sex- Call in sick to work one day. The night before, put a note into your honey's wallet/purse and ask them to meet you in the car at lunch for some midday brown-chicken-brown-cow. The next day, text your significant other and tell them to check their wallet/purse. Meet them at lunch and hump like two rats in a wool sock - except it will be in a car. FYI. Instead of a "sick day", tell your hunny bunny that you took a "Love Day"- bonus points for you, Eddy Haskell!

Psychology- Change up your morning routine. How many of you perform the same routine every damn morning? It's like a ritual or dance that we are performing awaiting death! Wake up, get into the shower. Clean your legs, arms, shampoo your hair...rinse. Dry off the same body parts. Check yourself out in the mirror. Shrug in disgruntlement. Brush your teeth. Dress yourself. Right leg, then left. Eat breakfast and then drive off in your car to work? How fucking depressing is that! Change it up! Wake up and walk around your house naked. Wave to your neighbor as you get the newspaper (naked if you please.) Listen to your favorite song in the shower, "A country boy can survive." At the very least, switch everything up so your brain isn't on auto pilot. Twenty percent of our daily energy is consumed by the brain. The more we challenge it, the more likely it is to stay spry.

Injuries- Medial and lateral elbow pain can be a bitch and very disabling. We need to determine if the pain is from overuse such as progression too fast or too heavy, or from a tight muscle either above or below the place of injury. Stand with your back and feet against a wall. Aim for keeping your back as flat against the wall as possible. Beginning with your arms at your side, slowly raise them above your head. If your back comes off the wall and arches, your lats (back) are tight. Place your hands on a high enough table and raise your arms above your head. Hold the stretch for 30 seconds.

Nutrition- Buy a scale. Not the kind I told you to shit on and throw away, I'm talking about a food scale. It will diligently teach you what the proper serving sizes are. Four to five ounces of meat is about the size of an average female's hand. Americans love to eat, that's no secret. Before we know it, we will be a bunch of fatasses like Gilbert Grape's mom unless we do something about it. A great first step would be measuring out your food and meals. Play some good ol' country, have a glass of wine, and use Sunday and Wednesday nights to cook up a storm. Nothing sexier than a girl in a Longhorns XL t-shirt cooking in her undies!

Exercise- Put $5 in a jar whenever you miss a workout (or however much you want Mr. /Mrs. $50 ballers). After the jar is full it doesn't mean you get to go buy a new pair of Lulu pants, not so fast Mr. /Ms. Flakster! Go to Starbucks and get yourself a black coffee (no treats for you fuckers because you slacked) and then give the rest to the barista. Tell the barista you want to donate the rest to the people in line. See, now you did something nice for someone else.

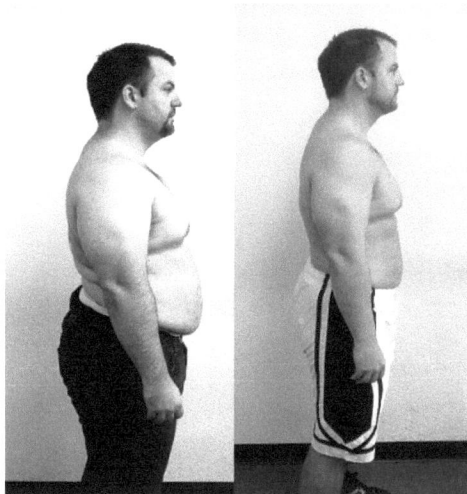

Client 5:

Beginning weight: 287lbs @ 31.8% body fat
Total S.P.I.N.E.™ score of 18

Results after 12 weeks:
239lbs @ 20.4% body fat (lost over 40lbs of fat)
Lost over 19 total inches
Total S.P.I.N.E.™ score of 27
Comments:
<u>Workouts:</u> "I was super surprised at how fast I started seeing results from the no grains. I liked how the workouts changed from phase to phase. In the beginning, I hated doing legs because mine were weak, especially my glutes! After three months, my legs ended up being my favorite muscle group to workout. Everything that Chris' says, truly works."
<u>Diet & Cheats:</u> "The first month trying to get rid of grains sucked- it wasn't easy, that's for damn sure. I slipped up, but when I did, I made sure to get right back on the no grain path. I did enjoy having the occasional cheat meal after a hard workout. My buddies and I would go get some pizza and I didn't feel bad or anything because I put the hard work in beforehand."
<u>Motivation:</u> "Be happy with who you are first and then create a vision for who you want to become. Live in the moment and be consistent and focused. Success is a planned event!"

I just had to put this one in, look how happy he is!

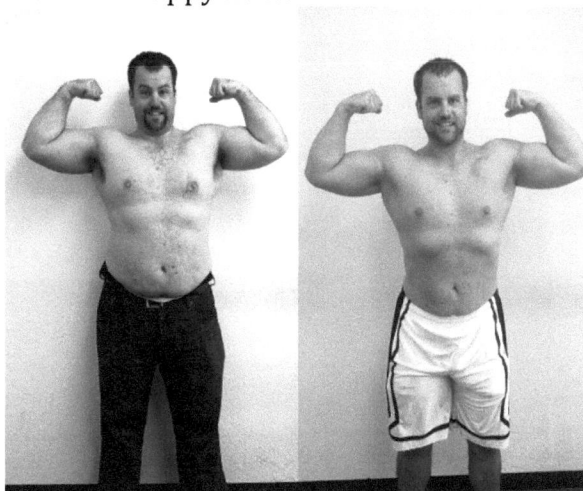

Chapter 7

S.P.I.N.E.™: What the fuck to do now

Holy Shit Factoid of the Day:
Did you know the average person's S.P.I.N.E.™ score increased 10.3 points for an average scale loss of 20.5 lbs in 12 weeks? Holy Fucking Shit the VTD does work!

I think I am part of a small population who cares about how things are done. I would be willing to bet two chupacabra dicks that my readers are more concerned with "when" it will be done. There may have been times when this information was a little over your head, and I apologize for that. I have to remember that your end goal isn't to become a certified personal trainer, it's to lose fat and become healthier.

The purpose of this book is to change how you think about and view fat loss. This ignorant nation believes it's only about nutrition or exercise. I highly disagree, which is why I created the acronym S.P.I.N.E.™. I believe we need to address: sex, stress, sleep, psychology and injuries as well. By following the 12 weeks of workouts and step-by-step diet plan, you will drastically change your S.P.I.N.E.™ score and be on the right path for eternal health. I know you have been "guaranteed" results before, hell, I did it in this book, but have you ever been deemed eternal health? That's one powerful fucking statement. Even in your afterlife you'll be fit! Match that one infomercial bitches!

What to Do Next
Now that you have read the book, you might be wondering which supplements to take. None. Don't waste your money on a bunch of chemicals. Pharmaceutical companies are just raping your ignorant assholes and it doesn't feel good. Drink your water, eat your fruits and veggies, stay away from grains, and follow my 12 weeks of workouts - you'll be fucking awesome if you just do just that.

The only suggestions I would make would be whey or vegan protein to supplement your nutrition if you're lacking protein. Ideally, I would like you to get your protein requirements through natural food sources, but, if you can't, buy some protein. I like Dreams First. It doesn't contain hormones and it only has seven ingredients.

If you do need energy have a good ol' cup of Joe, or some oatmeal and half an apple before you workout! Your money is far better spent on nutritious food. Granted, it's like telling a high school kid not to have sex, if you want to take something, be smart. With pre-workout supplements, do your research, start off with small doses, and be aware you will become super wired! Be sure to drink plenty of water and take it in cycles i.e., one or two weeks on then take a week off. Supplements are designed to get you hooked so you eventually become immune to it. You'll end up going back to the store in search of the newest and more expensive version. Don't come to Uncle Chris when you have a brain tumor or stroke, I will just say I told you so and ask to be in your will. The whole pre workout/supplement industry scares the holy fuck out of me. Way worse than the world's scariest movie: "I Know What You Did Last Summer". Fuck you, that movie was scary! I know, I am a big pussy when it comes to scary movies; that hook still gives me bad dreams!

Fix Your S.P.I.N.E.™

What do Jeanne Calment and Jack LaLanne have in common? Longevity. Jeanne lived to be 122 years old and Jack aka "The Godfather of Fitness" died at the age of 96. Jack was exercising until he died. Doctors say he could have lived longer if he would have stopped exercising through his pneumonia and just rested. Jeanne did what every young woman aspires to do: marry rich! At the age of 21, she married a wealthy store owner and never had to work a day after that. Seriously, she never had any stressors. She even fucking smoked! So what do these two have in common, their S.P.I.N.E.™ score was extremely high. Jack worked out all the time (literally) while Jeanne had zero life stressors. She enjoyed doing things she loved at no expense. The take-home story is if you want to live a healthy, long life: stress less, workout more, eat well, and keep on showing up. If your S.P.I.N.E.™ is healthy, you'll be too.

First Things First

Before you start fixing your S.P.I.N.E.™ and implementing these words, I want you to do three things:
1. Go have sex. Whatever pent up stuff you have in you right now is a part of the old you. Go get it out. A friend, booty call, ex, whatever, just do it. On to new and brighter things!
2. Close your eyes and imagine how you'll look three months from now. Your behavior will not change until you want it to. I have given you the proper tools to condition your bad behaviors of the past, but the choice for change is completely yours to dictate. Failure will not happen. Trust me. It's like the beloved "Peter Pan" movie with Robin Williams. Remember when he goes back to Never Never Land to rescue his kids? Before he is ready to face Captain Dildo, he has to recondition his mind by training with the Lost Boys. One night, they are all indulging in a festive dinner. Peter doesn't know what is going on because he can't imagine it. He finally realizes he lacked imagination - he couldn't see the food because he didn't believe in himself. He finally sees what everyone else has been seeing because he fully understands what it takes to succeed. It was there the whole time, he just couldn't see it! The same goes for your fat loss goals. The end goal is in sight and it's achievable. The question is, can you see it? If you're not mentally ready, how can you expect your body to change? Peter Pan analogy, check.
3. Show Up. Half the battle is showing up. Your past behavior and how you respond are going to be monumental. If you continue to walk down that old, disgusting beaten path, then you will continue to be fat, unhappy, and die an early death. Start by making the right choices and tell yourself that fatness no longer has control over you; you control your own destiny.

How You'll Succeed

If you gathered from this book that I am trying to make you look like a fitness model, you're smoking crack. I want you guys to be happy with your life. There will be no more Debbie Downer days of feeling like shit because you "cheated" and had a piece of cake. VTD is going to teach you how to get your best body by putting in the proper work. Together, we will fix your nutrition and exercise portion of the S.P.I.N.E.™ by taking grains out of your diet and replacing them with more fruits, vegetables, and water. Your energy levels will greatly increase because you're now working out 4-5 days a week. The SPI portion will increase from sleeping more and managing your stress. Sex will no longer be looked at as a chore. Your kids are going to need ear plugs because the new inner tiger/tigress will be unleashed and it's time for some rip roaring animal sex. More importantly, you will be in control of your actions and choices by understanding your behaviors are at the mercy of you. Your S.P.I.N.E.™ score is going to significantly increase by implementing the ways to fix your S.P.I.N.E.™ and following the workouts and nutrition plans. Additionally, here are some ways you will succeed.

1- Show Up. The biggest and best transformations that I have seen are from the people who have the highest adherence.

2- Subscribe to the VTD system for 30 consecutive days. I have been told by some clients that Paleo and/or Mediterranean diets are horrible. When asked how long they tried the diet for they responded by saying, "10 days"- that's a baboons cock! Stop looking for excuses why you're not succeeding and give it 100% effort for 30 days. After that, lambaste away. I personally guarantee if you follow everything I have said to a T (not a lower case t, a big fucking T) you will feel and look better than you did when you started.

3- Find a support group. You are who you surround yourself with. How many times have you told a family member or friend you're going on a diet and then all of a sudden they are encouraging you to have an extra piece of pie? Misery loves company, my VTDers, don't succumb to it. If your significant other isn't on board, tempt them with something like this, "Hunny, if you watch the kids for the next hour and cook dinner, I'll buy you tickets to that (enter whatever significant other likes) or I can just lick your asshole." Throw some chains or kinky shit in there; whatever works! Come on people; let's get excited for this shit.

4- Work hard. "I had one hell of a workout today" says the five-mile runner. No, you didn't. You just put a bunch of wear and tear onto your body and lowered your metabolism because you're burning muscle. Working hard is a relative term. These workouts will be hard and rewarding if followed properly.

5- Give up grains. See number 2. Additionally, I want to address counting calories. It's very challenging and if that's your style, have at it. ToneUp, an app that will help you determine daily calories was designed for consumers to see if predetermined goals are even realistic. Oh ya, ToneUp is an app that my student Tony and I made. With the help of one of my Show Up Clients, Satya, we were able to design (Satya) a bad-ass app. It will tell you how many calories and grams of protein that you need and it's easy to adjust on the fly. It's free to download, just make sure to leave us an awesome review.

6- Be human; life happens. The last thing I want you to feel is guilty due to the cookies and cream ice cream you just inhaled because your boss yelled at you. I want to teach you how to make proper choices and correct your behavioral patterns. If your boss is being a stinkhole, then go have a kick-ass workout. If you don't feel better by taking your aggression out in the gym, have that bowl of ice cream after. Hell, have two scoops. These opportune windows after resistance training are times when your muscles will soak up the carbs and signal your muscles to grow. Let's make smarter choices and learn to outsmart our body.

Pussy Chris Story
I don't want sympathy points, but when I was a sixth grader in elementary school, I had 48 sick days. I had bronchitis, allergic reactions to corn syrup which made me break out in hives, and giardia (parasite that gives you a massive case of the runs). My dad claims I was "milking it" and maybe I was - I was a clever little shit! I enjoyed staying at home. Who wouldn't love watching movies like "Peter Pan" and "Blank Check" while eating comfort foods all day long? I remember

vividly, my parents were fed up with my shenanigans and made me go back to school. My dad dropped me off at the backside of the school and I was bawling like I had just lost my favorite teddy bear, Poo Bear (that's a manly name for a teddy bear so shut the fuck up). Even though my dad told me everything was going to be alright, that walk to my classroom was the longest 200 yards ever! I was doing one of those belly cries. Looking back now, I was a huge pussy. I was scared to face the music. What if I had an asthma attack? What if I broke out in hives? What if I had explosive diarrhea and shit myself in the middle of class? Guess what happened? Nothing. I was afraid of the worst case scenario and nothing happened. I ended up having an awesome day! We talked about Lewis and Clark, picked our fantasy football teams (my teacher was a badass; she was way ahead of the times with the fantasy football shit!), played some basketball, and I think I even saw my first pair of tits! I will always remember those beautiful mountains for the rest of my life. She was wearing overalls and every time she bent over, I could get a side peak of them. I pitched a tent in my pants for a solid five minutes - man, I love boobies!

Why the fuck did I just lament about that stupid story? That little pussy kid back in sixth grade is you reading this right now. You're afraid of facing your worst fears because of what you think may happen. "I might fail", "what if I don't lose weight", "what if I hurt myself?" If I could've had my way, I would have stayed home forever and I bet I would have turned into one creepy fucking kid, that's for damn sure. I won't let that happen to you guys. You will succeed. You will lose fqt and if you follow everything that I have said, everything will turn out just as you imagined it. As in my story, everything will work out way better than you expect!

You have two options: show up or shut up. Hold yourself accountable and use the words in The Vulgar Truth Diet to help you take action. At the end of the day, it's going to be you who'll get these results; I'm just the helping hand. If you want to put a stop to this obesity epidemic, it begins with you. Now, I am challenging you to 100% complete the VTD, what are you going to do? It's time to put all the excuses and bullshit behind us; it's time to Show Up.

The End.

Inspiring quotes to live by:

You miss 100% of the shots you don't take. -Wayne Gretzky

Fall seven times and stand up eight. –Japanese Proverb

The way to get started is to quit talking and begin doing. –Walt Disney

I'd rather be a failure at something I enjoy than a success at something I hate. -George Burns

It's not the years in your life that count. It's the life in your years. –Abraham Lincoln

Insanity: doing the same thing over and over again and expecting different results. -Albert Einstein

Too many of us are not living our dreams because we are living our fears. –Les Brown

No man has the right to be an amateur in the matter of physical training. It is a shame for a man to grow old without seeing the beauty and strength of which his body is capable – Socrates

If a man tells a woman he loves the way she looks after sex, that's a bonus point. - Ava Cadell

The secret of getting ahead is getting started. -Mark Twain

Lack of activity destroys the good condition of every human being.
While movement and methodical physical exercise save it and preserve it. –Plato

Once you learn to quit, it becomes a habit. -Vince Lombardi

Physical fitness is not only one of the most important keys to a healthy body; it is the basis of dynamic and creative intellectual activity. - John F. Kennedy

For those who are given to excess, abstinence is easier than moderation – John Drybred.

You will get all you want in life if you help other people get what they want. – Zig Ziglar

Shallow men believe in luck. Strong men believe in cause and effect. - Ralph Waldo Emerson

Twenty years from now you will be more disappointed by the things that you didn't do than by the ones you did do, so throw off the bowlines, sail away from safe harbor, catch the trade winds in your sails. Explore, Dream, Discover. –Mark Twain

Sleep if the best meditation. – The Dalai Lama

Shake and Bake! – *Talladega Nights*

Nothing is impossible, the word itself says, "I'm possible!" –Audrey Hepburn

The time to repair the roof is when the sun is shining. - John F. Kennedy

I once wrestled an anaconda for 4 days, then realized I was masturbating – Chuck Norris poster

The best revenge is massive success. –Frank Sinatra

The doctor of the future will give no medicine but will interest his patience in the care. – Thomas Edison

Be the kind of person that when your feet hit the floor each morning the devil says - "Oh Fuck, there up!" - Not sure

Believe in yourself and all that you are. Know that there is something inside you that is greater than any obstacle. – Christian D. Larson

Eighty percent of success is showing up. –Woody Allen

Look well to the spine for the cause of disease – Hippocrates (Hippocrates could see into the future and knew I was going to invent S.P.I.N.E.™, luckily they didn't know how to trademark words back then!)

SHOW UP OR SHUT UP – Chris Hitchko

HORMONE INDEX

Hormone Super Heroes:

The study of hormones, aka endocrinology, is complex and fascinating. The combined weight of all the organs within this system is between 1-2 lbs. The system works by regulating bodily functions through glands, chemical substances, and a target organ - the Pituitary Gland releases LH (Luteinizing Hormone.) This hormone pinpoints the adrenal cortex to release Androgens which then takes aim at the testes which releases Testosterone. Hormones are "chemical messengers," affecting growth and behavior. Men and women produce the same hormones in different levels i.e., estrogen and testosterone - we produce both hormones. There are four broad categories of hormones: steroid, peptide, fatty acid compounds and amino acid derivatives. It's no longer calories in versus calories out; it's how the calories impact our hormones.

There are over 20 diseases related to obesity, by learning what the endocrine system does, you'll have a better chance of defeating them. I am going to explicate some hunger related hormones (Ghrelin, CCK and Leptin), the sleep hormone (Melatonin), some catabolic hormones (Cortisol, Glucagon & the Catecholamines) and then the Anabolic hormones (Testosterone, HGH, IGF's and Insulin.) There are many other hormones, however, they aren't that important regarding resistance training, i.e. Estrogen and Progesterone, which are very important for the development and maintenance of female sex characteristics (menstruation and reproductive cycles).

Now, let me introduce the Hormone Super Heroes; hormones that are affected by dieting and exercise.

Leptin - Aka "The Satiety Hormone" was just recently discovered in the early 1990s. Professors were harassing mice and discovered an important hormone released inside the fat cell responsible for satiety (fullness). It plays an important role in regulating energy intake and expenditure. Leptin travels from the fat sources throughout the body into the bloodstream, to the brain, and tells the hypothalamus "that's enough, or else we will be a big fat ass!" We aren't 100% sure if Leptin either suppresses appetite or if it reduces chemicals that stimulate hunger. As with Insulin, continuous overexposure may result in Leptin resistance. In other words, the fatter you are, the larger amounts of Leptin you'll have floating around because the brain no longer recognizes it – we don't know when to stop eating!

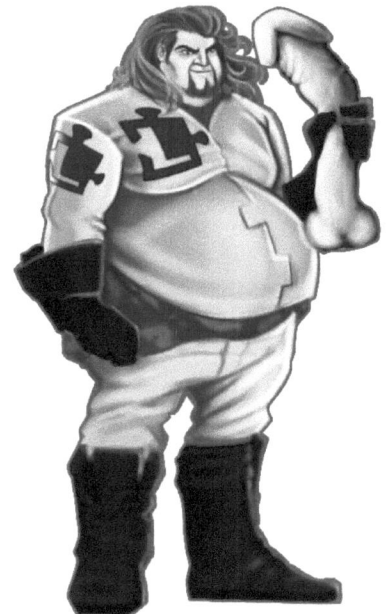

So what is our society doing to fix this physiological mess? Mandate exercise as part of our daily routines? HAHA, yeah right! How can the government make money off our simple souls if they suggested this? Pharmaceutical companies are trying to synthesize compounds that mimic the lost result of satiety. Here lies a huge problem: we are continuously trying to fix our chubby ass habits by popping more pills. This won't work. It's going to take a behavioral change. Follow VTD and do it the natural way.

Ghrelin - Aka Mr. Gremlin is released from the stomach and makes us hungry. In the morning, Ghrelin is at its highest. Throughout the day, when its concentration is low, you're not

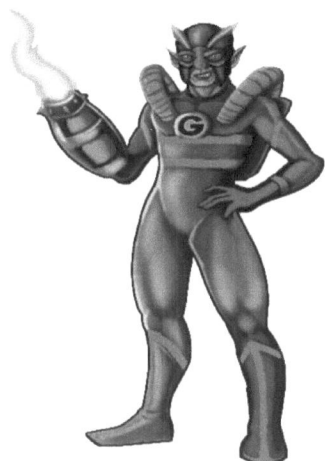

hungry. Besides being known as the hunger hormone, it can also raise the levels of HGH. This is one of the reasons we encourage one day of fasting per week during the third part of the nutrition plan. What is the favorite excuse why people don't eat breakfast? "I'm not hungry!" Well, nincompoop, you are hungry; unfortunately, you have conditioned yourself to ignore the signal. It's important to note that I suggest not skipping breakfast as a beginner in a new program. Sorry, but you're mentally weak and can't handle the lower blood sugar levels - you're going to become enervated, shake a little bit, and all of a sudden smash a box of Oreos! Studies have shown that you're more likely to be overweight if you habitually skip breakfast, so don't. After two months of this system, you'll be conditioned and prepared to handle it. It will be a shock to your system as you follow my suggestions and experience the results!

Cholecystokinin (CCK) - A hormone produced by the duodenum (first foot of the small intestine) and released in the brain in response to the presence of fats and proteins. CCK causes the contraction of the gallbladder, release of bile, and secretion of pancreatic digestive enzymes. It's the principal stimulus for delivery of pancreatic enzymes and bile into the duodenum to secrete the proper digestive enzymes. Increased blood levels of CCK can be found 15-20 minutes after a meal and can remain elevated up to three hours. Kind of boring, but look at the drawing with three boobs! BOOBIES!

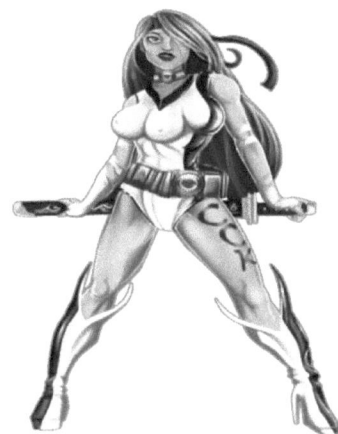

Melatonin - Melatonin is a hormone produced by the pineal gland (small gland in the brain) as a response to darkness. This is why it's important to limit the exposure

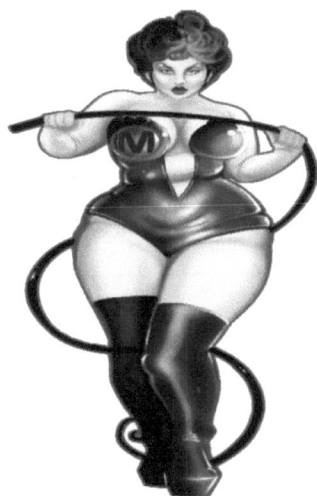

to light before bed. If you're constantly surrounded by light (TV, phones and/or computers), your brain won't release your sleep hormone! The body has a natural internal clock that controls sleep, aka circadian rhythms. I suggest a minimum of eight hours of sleep, but some say they can get by on six. "Getting by" is way different from proper functioning. If I have been drinking, I can get by on four hours of sleep if I wake up and keep drinking. The point is, I don't want y'all to just "get by" with sleep. It's imperative to get enough sleep or your pudgy midline will stick around. If you truly want to know how your internal clock works, go camping for a week without any alarm clocks. When you go to sleep, your natural sleeping cycle would be when you wake up. Use that excuse for your next few days off, "Hey Mr. Bossman. I am gonna need to take the next week off to see what my normal sleep cycles are!" HA, wouldn't that be awesome if they agreed!

Catabolic - Breakdown

All hormones have their role, but let's make it clear; there are no bad hormones. Hormones are like sex; healthy in good amounts and depressing in smaller ones. If you get laid regularly and indiscriminately, you could get an STD and die. Maybe a little extreme, but you get the point. Not enough or too much is painful; we need just the right amount.

Cortisol – This "fight or flight" hormone is produced during times of stress and low blood sugar from the adrenal cortex (small gland on top of the kidneys). Its main function is to yield glucose for working muscles through gluconeogenesis (the generation of new glucose molecules by way of non-carbohydrate substrates: protein, fat, and other byproducts of exercise). Long duration and high intense exercise produce the greatest amounts of cortisol i.e. 60+ minutes of cardio and/or crossfit-like intense workouts. During long duration and/or high intense exercise, Cortisol levels may remain elevated for up to two hours. It serves as an antagonist (opposite) to insulin, which inhibits glucose uptake. Hence the importance to spike the hell out of your blood sugar levels immediately after exercise to mitigate the effects of Cortisol by elevating insulin levels. Think of Cortisol being afraid of insulin after a workout. Serum concentrations are usually elevated in the morning and dissipate throughout the day. Another reason to implement intermittent fasting is to maximize lipolysis (fat burning) by not eating breakfast. Eating a breakfast rich in carbohydrates such as cereal, a bagel with cream cheese and/or a breakfast sandwich turns the body's fat storing mechanism on instead of maintaining a fat-burning environment – no bueno! Cortisol is also produced in copious amounts during times of chronic stress i.e. divorce, lack of sleep, war, studying for finals, and endurance related activities. So, stop worrying, Cortisol will break down your muscles, connective tissue, lower immunity, and increase fat storage around the midsection. This is why many endurance athletes have a spare tire. They produce a shit ton of cortisol during their event – consequently, storing fat around the stomach. The same can be said for women and menopause. During this time, usually around age 50, there is a reduction of estrogen and progesterone (another important female hormone that is crucial for the regulation of menstruation). Best ways to limit your exposure to high amounts of C is to de-stress i.e., sleep 8-10 hours and stop being a fucking grumpasorus - just be happy! Adrenal fatigue, which can be caused from stressing all the time, can causes an inverse relationship with your normal C levels. When C levels are elevated at night and low in the morning, intervention is needed. Your glands are working overtime therefore, lethargy, fat storage and overtraining is likely.

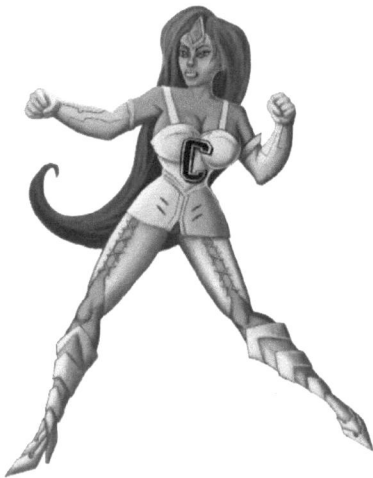

Glucagon –Glucagon elevates blood sugar levels by increasing the release of glucose into the body through stored glycogen in the liver when blood sugar levels become low. A diet low in carbs, prolonged exercise, and/or starvation stimulates the release of Glucagon via the alpha-cells of the pancreas. There isn't much of a response during exercise because Cortisol and the Catecholamine's are doing the majority of the work. That's it.

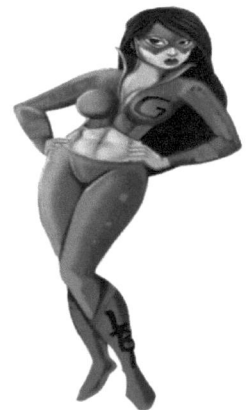

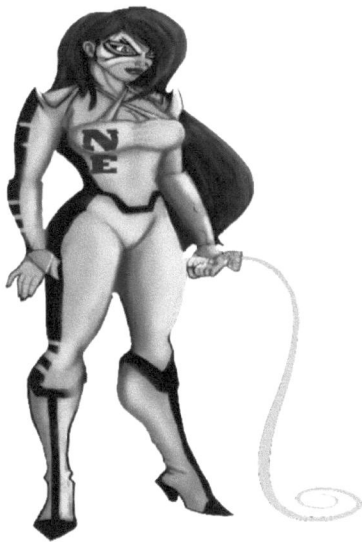

Epinephrine & **Norepinephrine** – Also known as the "fight or flight hormones" and with the addition on Dopamine, they are commonly referred to as Catecholamines. The main functions of Epinephrine and Norepinphrine respectively are glycogenolysis and lipolysis (breakdown glycogen and fat) for immediate energy in times of stress. Remember, exercise is a form of stress. When you answer the door and you see a 500 lb. Silverback gorilla, your choices are to either fight the big hairy ass mother fucker or put your tail between your legs and run like hell! Either way, you will instantaneously increase blood sugar levels for instant energy usage. If you want to do a quick, very fun test, do the following. Yell out "AHHHHHHH" at the top of your lungs and watch people freak out. You can tell them you were just checking their fight or flight responses - no biggie, they'll live.

Anabolic – Build Up

These suckers are all powerful hormones that build tissue. All hormones function in their respected manner in the right amount. Too little or too much of any of these hormones can have negative long-term effects, so take caution. If you are going to try something crazy and take one, chat with your doctor and try to have your organs and blood levels checked so nothing bad happens. If your body is already functioning properly, by not cycling on and off, you can permanently destroy your organs!

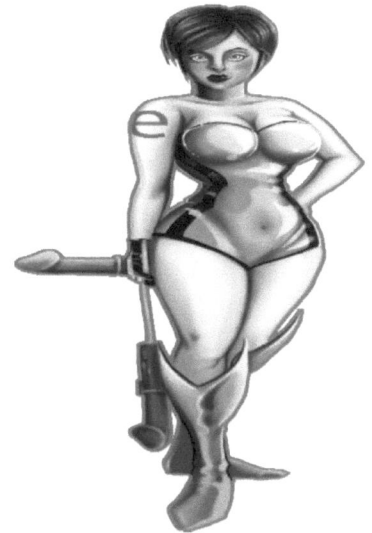

Testosterone – T is released from the testes in males and ovaries in females. There are many effects of Testosterone including: stimulates the development of sex characteristics (deepening of the voice, hair, muscle tonus), increases energy, libido, and increases muscle and bone growth. *Cholesterol is the precursor to this hormone (and all steroid hormones) - so stop ordering egg whites. That's an old myth and you need the yolk for proper T production, and it has 13 essential nutrients! T levels are highest in the morning, hence morning wood. The reference range for normal T for males is between 300 – 1000 and females between 20-70 ng/dl (nanograms per deciliter). The range in my opinion is donkey shit because of the ambiguity. I lost a $50 bet to my roommate because my T levels were in the low 400s while he had over 500. Why can't I supplement and be up to his level - cry me a river, Chris! The best ways to increase your T levels is to sleep properly, exercise with heavier weights, and avoid beer, soy, and stress.

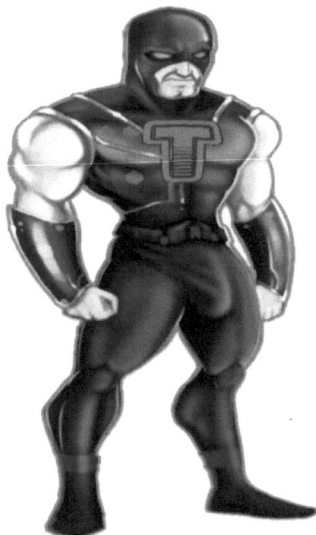

To maximize the release of testosterone during a workout, it's best to shoot for 1-5 reps (max effort of 85-100% of your 1 rep max) with longer rest periods (greater than 3 minutes). Obviously, the best way to increase T is to do 'roids. Just be careful because how do you really know what is in that tiny, little vial? Sodium? Water? Urine? Who knows! Guys, if you want to turn into a girl, take Estrogen. Girls, if you want to turn into a guy, take T. It's not rocket science, give the opposite sex the main key that separates the sexes and you'll turn into that sex.

*What are the benefits of cholesterol you be asking? Here we are: essential component of our cell membranes, necessary for digestion, fertility, brain development, and functioning. Cholesterol is also essential for the synthesis of bile (breaks down fats) and vitamin D from the sunlight. 75% of Cholesterol is synthesized in many body tissues (mainly the liver, but also skin, testes, ovaries, adrenal cortex, and intestines), and 25% comes from the diet.

Human Growth Hormone – Produced by the hypothalamus, this potent hormone stimulates tissue growth and metabolism. It also stimulates the release of IGF-1&2 which increases protein synthesis. The three great ways to maximize the release of GH are through deep sleep, high intense exercise, and times of fasting. This hormone is released in large quantities during puberty. So, the next time you start yelling at your teenager for sleeping too much, you need to muzzle it because sleep is needed to grow! Hypo-secretion of this hormone results in dwarfism aka Mini Me.

VTD suggests sleeping between 8-10 hours nightly. In week three, we introduce high intense intervals and in the third part of the diet we suggest intermittent fasting. See, there is a reckoning for my madness; it's to maximize the release of HGH! When taken exogenously in large amounts (inorganically by way of shots), it can grow bodily organs. Ever wonder why many body builders have protruding stomachs yet still have a dialed in 6-pack? That's a sign that HGH is being used: their organs have grown. You may feel great, but do you think it's normal for the intestines to grow? No judgments, just a simple question. I am not afraid of body builders because guess what the best defense is? Run like you were just caught watching *Girls* on HBO. Not only does their cardio usually suck baboons ass, but their tendons are prone to snap because they are so freakin' huge! To maximize the release of growth hormone during a workout, it's best to aim between 10+ reps and rest periods of less than a minute.

Insulin-Like Growth Factors (IGFs) - Produced by the liver, this anti-catabolic, growth-promoting hormone is released through stimulation of HGH. As with HGH, its main role is proliferation of skeletal cells, but also has effect on bone, cartilage, kidneys, skin, lungs, and nerves. To maximize the release of this hormone, make sure to get proper amounts of sleep, and during exercise, aim for larger muscles with shorter rests (squats for 8-10 reps, rest for a minute and repeat for 5 sets). FYI, putting a deer antler up your ass isn't going to get you all big and bulky. You would need to have like 100 antlers and scrape all the velvet from them to get stronger, faster, and bigger. Stop looking for quacky ways to get large. Put in the required work in the gym for a couple years and then weigh your decisions.

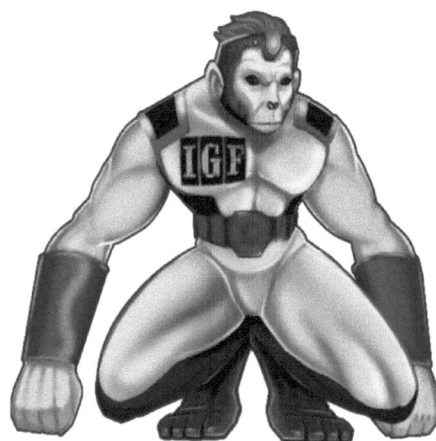

Insulin – This hormone is the *Jersey Shore* of hormones. Non-Insulin dependent diabetes aka Type II diabetes is all over the news because of the obesity epidemic. This type of diabetes is preventable, whereas type I (aka insulin dependent or juvenile diabetes) is seen in less than 5-10% of people with diabetes. Insulin is produced by the pancreatic beta-cells and shuttles glucose into specialized cells called glucose transporters aka GLUTs. When blood sugar levels rise, insulin is released to absorb the sugar.

Imagine a 30x30 classroom with 50 students (insulin) sitting at desks with seat belts on. Picture a group of magical balloons dropping from the ceiling (the balloons symbolize sugar after being digested and absorbed by the small intestine). An alarm sounds unbuckling "X" amount of students' seat belts; the release of more balloons will correlate with the release of more students i.e., a candy bar would release 50 students whereas an apple would release 20. The students' job is to pick up a balloon and bring it to door at the front of the classroom. Each student has a magical key to unlock the door. Once the door is open, there is a specialized UPS worker aka GLUT transport who then takes the balloon from the student to use immediately as energy, or takes it away to store in the muscles or fat.

If glycogen is depleted, usually after a workout and with active individuals, glucose will be stored in the muscle. Otherwise, the UPS worker will take the balloons to the dumpster to be turned into fat (sugar consumption makes us fat, not fat intake). It's important to note that there are technically several UPS workers and they all respond differently (14, but more will probably be discovered with newer technologies). To maximize absorption of glucose, resistance training needs to be the primary exercise.

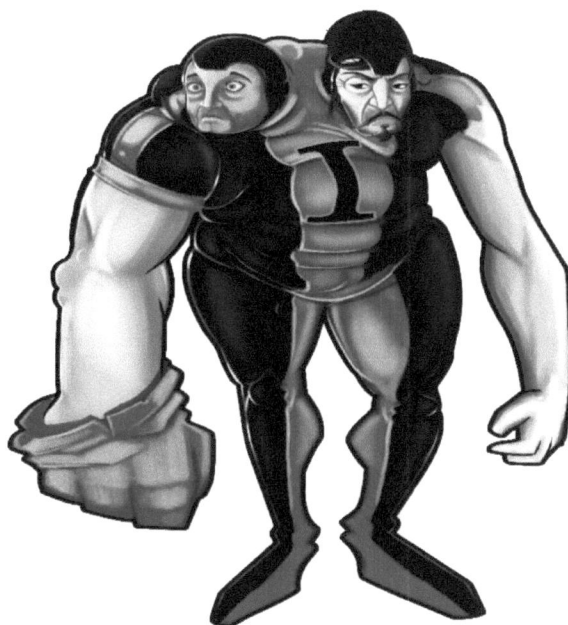

Now to better understand type II diabetes, let's use the same example. The students in the classroom are now noncompliant, fat, over 21, and have been drinking booze all day long! When the balloons are released into the room, they won't and cannot pick up the balloons to carry them to the door because they're fucking hammered (insulin resistance)! The brain does a role call to check and balance the internal system, but it registers a shit ton of balloons (sugar) so it releases more students (insulin). Essentially, the sugar is not removed and we are left with cells that cannot uptake the glucose. We are left with a heart disease, high blood pressure, kidney disease, blindness, amputation, and more than 200 billion dollars in total costs. All of this can be mitigated by implementing this system of eating properly, exercising regularly, and stopping day drinking, you drunken fucks!

It's important to at least have 1 day of rest. No pain, No gain isn't always the best adage. If your body is in pain, super sore or compromising sleep, take a day or two off and just adhere to a no grain diet.

www.ingramcontent.com/pod-product-compliance
Lightning Source LLC
Chambersburg PA
CBHW060808270326
41928CB00002B/26